I'm Still Here

I'm Still Here

A Memoir

Martina Reaves

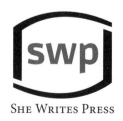

SHE WRITES PRESS

Published 2020
Printed in the United States of America
ISBN: 978-1-63152-876-7
ISBN: 978-1-63152-877-4
Library of Congress Control Number: 2019911280

For information, address:
She Writes Press
1569 Solano Ave #546
Berkeley, CA 94707

She Writes Press is a division of SparkPoint Studio, LLC.

To
My wife Tanya Starnes
and
Our son Cooper Reaves

CONTENTS

THE END OF THE LINE

It's the summer of 1969, uncommonly hot, no fog with a glaring sun. The air is still, like summer in New York or Chicago, but not San Francisco's usual June weather.

I wear yellow sandals and a very short shift, shocking pink with yellow stripes, which I made myself from a Simplicity pattern. On the corner of 18th and Sanchez, where I live in a flat with my high school friend Cindy, I see the J Church streetcar a block ahead. The driver rings the bell, and I run hard, making it just before the doors whoosh shut.

I settle into an old, worn, army-green seat and look out the window. Funky, decrepit Victorian buildings line the street on both sides. "Market Street!" the driver calls out. The streetcar slowly makes its way downtown. Third. Kearny. Geary. The next stop is mine. I'm headed to work.

"Greyhound Information, Miss Reaves," I purr into my headset. "How may I help you?" I try to make work fun by messing around with different voices. Last month, after two years at Pomona College, I decided to move to San Francisco and transfer to Cal for my junior year. Fortunately, I landed a summer job at Greyhound that pays $500 a month: enough for rent, food, clothing, entertainment, and then some. I feel prosperous and free.

"The next bus leaves for Sacramento at 3 p.m.," I tell the person on the other end of the line, "and then they leave every hour on the hour

1

until 8 p.m." I make a game out of the job. How many calls can I take in an hour? Once, I get to eighty.

I'm off work at 9:45 p.m. By then, the fog has rolled in and I stand at First and Market, shivering in my summer clothes until the J Church streetcar arrives. I haven't lived in the City long enough to know I should never leave the house without layers.

The driver has long blond hair. He wears a paisley scarf and next to his foot is a metal lunch box painted in bright psychedelic colors. Seated directly behind him is a Japanese woman, leaning forward with a straight back, a small, white, perfectly folded handkerchief in her hands. From time to time, she pats it against her smooth, pale face as she speaks slowly to the driver in Japanese. Intrigued, I watch from across the aisle.

I look for the streetcar driver again the next night, but no luck. Then, five nights later, he appears again, with the same lunch box, the same paisley scarf, this time with a satchel of books. Because there's nobody else in the car, I sit up front and ask him about his interest in Japanese. "I lived in Japan," I tell him. "My father was in the Navy, and we were stationed there. It's where I graduated from high school."

His name is David. "My friend Yoshiko is teaching me Japanese while I help her with English," he says. "I'm getting an MA at San Francisco State in Teaching English as a Foreign Language." Since I'm an Asian Studies major, we have lots to talk about.

"Eighteenth and Church," he calls out, and I jump off and run home to my flat a block away.

I soon learn that he drives the J line by my stop two nights a week just after I get off work. After several weeks of chatting, David asks me to stay on board and have tea with him at the end of the line at 30th and Church. A ritual develops: I join him twice a week for tea and we talk about our lives, Japan, music, books. He appeals to me in so many ways: his long, lanky looks, our Japan connection, his mind. He's older, of course. I peg him at twenty-nine or thirty, which would be a *little* old for me, but not enough to deter me. Because of his age, most likely, he's different. He really listens to me when we talk and takes my ideas seriously.

"My son is coming to live with me," David tells me over tea at the end of the line one night.

"Tell me about him," I say, trying to sound casual. I can't believe he has a child that I didn't know about!

"He's fifteen and wants to live with me instead of his mother. But my life isn't set up for him. I live in a studio. Everything will need to change." In my head, I quickly do the math. David must be at least thirty-five. I'm a little stunned and disappointed.

I get off the streetcar at 18th and Church and walk home. My roommate Cindy is with our neighbors, John and Ron, in their downstairs flat. We think they're gay, but it's never discussed.

Holding my hand to my brow, I walk in their door and throw my vintage red velvet coat across the room. "My streetcar driver has a fifteen-year-old son!" I wail.

The boys laugh and ask me a few questions. "I've been riding on his streetcar for weeks, twice a week. We talk. I've had my eye on him."

"What's his name?" Ron asks.

"David Patton."

"Oh, my God! I know about him! I just read about him in the *Chronicle* this morning." Ron runs from the room and returns with the newspaper. "Listen to this! Your streetcar driver not only has a son! He's an Episcopal priest!" He reads an excerpt from Herb Caen's column. Herb thinks it's funny that a priest drives the J Church streetcar looking like a hippie.

Reeling, I pull out David's phone number from my huge canvas purse and go up to our flat to call him. It's the first time we've ever talked by phone, but I have to know the truth.

"I hate people to know I'm a priest," he says when I tell him I saw the story, "because once they know, they never treat me the same. I have a little church on Mission where I preach on Sundays, but it's part-time work. I'm mostly out of the church now, since I got divorced."

I'm both surprised by the news and relieved that he's finally opening up more about his life. We've talked a lot about our current lives, but not much about the past.

The next time I see him, I get on his streetcar after work at 9:45. He invites me to come home with him, so I ride with him until the end of his shift at midnight. His studio is a small space on Octavia just off Market Street, sparsely furnished with a single bed, a music stand, a rug, a violin, and lots of books: cookbooks, poetry collections, and school texts. In the minuscule kitchen, his macrobiotic grains and vegetables are lined up, tidy and efficient. It's like a monk's cell.

I sit on the single bed, the only space available, and within minutes we're making love.

TONGUE

It's 2008 and I'm pacing around our kitchen, talking with Tanya, my partner of twenty-eight years. She's lounged in a chair, her blue eyes on me, her compact body agitated. "We have to let Cooper know," I say. "There's too much risk he'll hear from someone else."

"Let's give him a few more days," she says.

Cooper is our twenty-two-year old son, who's in his final year of college studying sustainable development in Costa Rica. Day after day, we wait for him to call because we want him to be the one to initiate contact. It's part of our letting-him-go process. Finally, though, we send an email telling him we need to talk.

He calls on Skype, his big, brown eyes and sweet, inquisitive face peering at us from the call center in San Jose. "What's up?" he asks.

"I have tongue cancer," I blurt. He flinches.

"How do you know?" he asks.

I give him the details: I'd gone to my doctor to get antibiotics for a chest infection and asked her to check a painful sore on my tongue.

"Hmmmm," she said. "I'd ask your dentist to look at it."

My dentist told me to get a biopsy, just to be sure. That word—biopsy—had jolted me.

A few days later, I sat in a fancy dental chair while an oral surgeon plucked out a small piece of my tongue to send to UCSF for analysis.

Then, we waited for results.

Finally, after three long days, the oral surgeon called to say

I had cancer, though I have no memory of this call: no memory of where I was, who was there, what I said in response. I must have been numb. After hearing the word "biopsy," my mind had replayed the summer of 1986 like a second-rate movie that wouldn't stop.

May 28, 1986, is one of those rare, crystalline days that Berkeley gets in the spring. Light dances on the budding leaves. The air feels almost tropical. I stand on the steps in front of Herrick Hospital on the Friday of my last day of maternity leave. Tanya is at home with three-month old Cooper. I've been feeling fuzzy-brained, feverish, and exhausted, but nobody can find anything wrong with me.

"You're just a new mother," my OB said. "This is normal."

My acupuncturist pronounced my qi excellent.

My dentist said my teeth are fine.

But something's wrong. I know it. I've considered mono, a wacky thyroid, or walking pneumonia.

This morning, I returned to my primary care doctor. "You've got to come up with an answer," I said. "I can't think straight. I keep having fevers. I can't go back to work Monday feeling like this, and I can't call in and say I'm not coming back if I don't know what's wrong with me."

She checked me out for the second time in a month, and in exasperation, sent me here for a chest X-ray.

Inside the hospital I step into a dark room. Put on a loose hospital gown. Scrunch my shoulders forward into a machine. Breathe in. Hold. Whirr. Click. It's done.

I wait in the hallway for my results. "There's something in your chest the size of a grapefruit," the radiologist says when he emerges. He doesn't look me in the eye. "We need to get a piece of it to find out what it is. Let me see what I can set up."

"What could it be?" I ask, so naïve I can only imagine a cyst or something like that.

"It could be a benign tumor; could be cancer; could be a cyst. We don't know. That's why we need to get a piece of it."

He shows me the X-ray. And there it sits. An octopus-like growth trying to strangle my heart. On the screen, it's bright white. I panic. My fingers shake as I dial our number from the dilapidated phone booth in the hallway. "I think you'd better come," I tell Tanya. "Something's wrong."

She leaves Cooper with our neighbor, and by the time she arrives at the hospital, the doctor is sticking a long needle with little pincers into my chest. It comes back empty.

"We'll have to schedule surgical biopsy," he says.

Three days later, on the Monday I was supposed to go back to work, I awake from the anesthetic for the biopsy to Dr. Yee's face, three inches from mine.

"Congratulations," he says, grinning. "You have the good kind of cancer."

I didn't know there was such a thing as "good" cancer. In fact, I don't know anyone my age who has even had cancer. What he means, I soon learn, is that the lymphoma in my chest is fast-growing and will respond well to chemotherapy.

Within twenty-four hours, after I get over the initial shock, I enter a strange state of euphoria. I'm calm; everything is clear. I know I won't be going back to my family law practice anytime soon; that this cancer is not going to kill me; that my life will go on. My sense of well-being is so profound that for days I float through life feeling at ease, even joyful.

This isn't to say there aren't grueling moments over the next three months. Horrifying procedures. Doctors, sweat dripping from their faces, sticking needles into my chest to drain fluids, while I watch on a monitor as my heart recoils whenever a needle gets too close. Weaning Cooper months before I had planned to in order to protect him from the drugs that will invade my body. Gruesome, debilitating chemotherapy dripping into my veins. Shaving my head when my hair starts to fall out. Hospitalization with pneumonia while our friends move us into our new house.

But through it all, I have an absolute conviction that I will survive. I do visualizations: little piranhas swim through my bloodstream gobbling up cancer cells; a luminous Mother Fish floats around me, watching over things, protecting me. I'm surrounded by Tanya, Cooper, and our friends—nourished and supported as I devote myself to saving my life.

"What does this mean? Tongue cancer," Cooper wants to know. "Are you hurting? Is it bad?"

"Right now, I'm mostly okay," I say. "I have stitches in my tongue where they took the biopsy, and it hurts a little, but not a lot. Later in the week, I'm getting a CT scan to see whether the cancer has spread down into my neck. We'll know more after that. Call us Friday and we'll fill you in."

When we hang up, I'm in tears. Cooper is just about to launch himself. My sweet, smart, passionate son. A man of almost twenty-two, with bits of the boy still clinging to him. I don't want my cancer to suck him back into the nest. I want him to soar.

On Friday the doctor tells Tanya and me that the CT scan looks clear. We're limp with relief, barely able to drive home. Cooper anxiously calls fifteen minutes early. "I brought my friend Emily with me for support." That's my boy, taking care of himself. "What did the doctor say?"

"It hasn't spread down my neck."

"Does this mean I don't have to stop my studies?"

"Honey, you don't need to change a thing. I'm going to be okay."

I tell him I'm having surgery in a week or so, then radiation. I don't tell him that this time, I'm scared.

"I'm really sorry this is happening," he says, "but I'm glad I don't need to come home. I really like this program."

I ache inside all around my heart.

After my first cancer diagnosis, I realized almost right away that I couldn't go back to my work as a family lawyer. For five years, I'd experienced tremendous inner conflict about the work I was doing. I'd felt cut off from myself, from my heart, from my spirit. I came to believe that a divorce is more complicated and nuanced than the adversarial system can handle, that pitting one side against the other doesn't make sense in most cases. After I got well, I couldn't bear the thought of representing one person against another. In fact, for a while I thought I'd never be a lawyer again. Then, little by little, I realized there were aspects of practicing law that I enjoyed: solving problems; thinking things through; drafting agreements; working intimately with people. It occurred to me that I could enjoy these things if I were a mediator, if I worked with a couple in a divorce to reach a resolution that made sense to both of them.

I found a mediation training I wanted to go to at Green Gulch, a conference center north of San Francisco. The trainer opened the workshop by asking the group of twenty aspiring mediators the following question: "What draws you to this work?"

Everyone had a story. I told mine: I was thirty-eight. I lived with my partner, Tanya, and our one-year-old, Cooper. I had a house and a law degree and was contemplating what to do with my life after cancer. As I shared, I felt teary and vulnerable, not at all lawyer-like. I figured I was in the right place.

During a break from the training, I walked down to Muir Beach with other classmates, through the abundant organic gardens, the salty air, the brisk wind. Sally, another student, looked at me with big, innocent eyes.

"Do you have any idea," she asked, "what you did to create that cancer?"

Even though I was used to people asking unbelievably offensive questions about my cancer, this one slammed me. I bit my tongue and thought fast. What I *wanted* to say was: "How stupid can you be? I didn't *create* my cancer. What I did was get born, live my life, and have some bad luck." What I *actually* said was: "I think cancer is complicated. It's a result of many things: genes, toxins in the air and in our food, stress. Who knows?" Then I immediately turned my attention to someone else to avoid more talk.

Aside from this interaction, the training was momentous for me. After five days, I came home inspired, excited, engaged. I printed up cards that said: MARTINA REAVES, ATTORNEY/MEDIATOR. I sent a letter to everyone in my Rolodex announcing that my practice would be limited to mediation. My new work required me to sink into the heart of things. To work deeply with people who were divorcing. To understand both sides. To try to resolve disputes. I learned that I could be myself as a mediator, that I could use the aspects of myself that I liked—empathy, connection, problem-solving. I no longer had to be a gladiator.

THE COMMUNE

At the end of the summer of 1969, David and I are sitting under fluorescent lights on red stools at the Formica counter in the little café at 30th and Church, drinking Lipton tea, the only choice, with milk. Since spending our first night together, we have a new ritual: we spend the night together on the two nights a week that he's on the J line. But we don't talk on the phone or go on real dates—he has no time for dates, being a full-time student, a full-time streetcar driver, and a part-time priest.

"I've found a six-bedroom house to rent in Diamond Heights up on Twin Peaks," he says. "It's in the middle of the city so I can get to any streetcar line for work. I'm going to start a commune."

"Why a commune?" I ask.

"It'll be better for my son to have other people around." He names the other people he's asking to move in: his son, of course; Bill Segen, another streetcar driver we both know; Ramesh, Bill's Indian friend; and two of David's other friends. "You want to live with me?" he asks.

By my calculations, all the bedrooms are taken, so I guess in a roundabout way he's asking me to share a bedroom with him. Curious, I go with him to see the house. It's an almost-new Eichler home, with radiant floor heating, a novel feature in 1969, two inner courtyards, a big kitchen and living room, all very modern. He shows me the master bedroom, which has its own bath at the far end of the house away from the street. "What do you think?" he asks.

"I'll think about it," I say.

"This is too weird," I tell Cindy when I get home the next morning. "I like him, he likes me, but we've never discussed love or anything about commitment, and now he wants me to live with him! What do I do? I'm not ready for this."

"Do you love him?"

"I think so."

"Then you've got nothing to lose. If you don't like it, you can move out. You'll pay a lot less rent, too. Why not try it?"

Here's what holds me back. David and I have never talked about our feelings for each other. We have fun, talk, make love, share meals, but "I love you" has never passed our lips. Not once. I can't move in with a man who doesn't even love me. I don't need marriage. I'm not even *interested* in marriage. But I want something more than simple convenience.

The next night, he asks me if I've had time to think about moving in. I ask him about his feelings and he mumbles about how hard feelings are. "What happens to me," he says, "is if I say how I'm feeling, the feeling goes away. If I'm feeling like I love you, I want to enjoy the feeling. I don't want to say it and make it go away." But a little later, he says, with conviction, "I love you," and for me, the deal is sealed. We move in together on October 1, 1969.

The folks in our household commit to a year. Ramesh becomes chief chef while he waits for his green card. There's always a spicy pot of chai tea on the stove, scenting the house with cinnamon, honey, nutmeg, and exotic spices I've never heard of. David's son, referred to as Little David even though he's well over six feet tall, arrives from Greenwich, Connecticut, where his long hair, beads, and hippie attire have been entirely unwelcome. He fits right into San Francisco. He and I try to peacefully co-exist, but it's strange being closer in age to him than David. I definitely don't feel like a parent, and he doesn't want me to parent. Little David would rather have his father to himself, so there's always a slight undercurrent of tension. Bill Segen changes jobs from streetcars to cable cars and comes home every night with a starry-eyed tourist who spends the night and is never seen again. It's the '60s, after all.

I attend UC Berkeley for exactly one week. When my advisor tells me that an Asian Studies major can't take a painting class, I leave his cramped office, take AC transit across the bridge and Muni back home, and I never return. Even though I've never studied art, I want to paint more than I want to study Chinese history in airless jam-packed classrooms. I keep my job at Greyhound and sign up for painting and sociology classes in San Francisco. I make abstracts of trees with bright colors that are four feet by six feet and bring them home on Muni to adorn the walls of our commune.

TALKING IS HIGHLY OVERRATED

On Valentine's Day 2008, the surgeon removes one-sixth of my tongue, ending all the way back into my tonsils. "Just let your tongue heal," he says. "No talking or chewing for two weeks. Eat liquids: soups, smoothies, yogurt."

Notebooks are scattered all over the house so I can communicate in writing with Tanya and my friends. Toward the end of my silent time, I flip through them. Some entries are mundane:

"I'm gonna get dressed so we can walk."

"Went to the loony bin and fell in love." This in response to a story about a friend of a friend who met her new boyfriend at a psychiatric hospital.

"Tea? Wine? A Manhattan?" Offerings to our friend Marjorie.

"It's easier to love them from afar." Comments about college-age sons.

Some entries are serious:

"I had a huge meltdown over the medical establishment." This had to do with communication with doctors and their assistants after I'd sent an email to my surgeon requesting information:

"Can I drink hot beverages now?"

"Can I chew a little if it doesn't hurt?"

"Is the appointment time I got with the radiologist soon enough?"

In response, an assistant had written back: "Try not to worry. You're in good hands. Relax." Not *one* question was answered. I couldn't talk, but sounds I'd never made in my life came out of my mouth. Not words, but deep-from-the-gut sounds. I jabbed all the words inside me onto the notebook: "THEY ARE PATRONIZING ME. THIS EMAIL TREATS ME LIKE I'M CRAZY AND NEUROTIC!!! MY QUESTIONS ARE LEGITIMATE!!!!!"

But as I live these two weeks without the spoken word, I realize that talking is *highly* overrated. There are far too many words that just fill space, unnecessary, unimportant words that don't pierce the heart of things.

A lot of the time, my mind simply drifts in the silence.

One morning, I have a thought as I awaken: I've been biting my tongue so long it finally bit back! Then my mind floats to a life-sized ceramic sculpture I once made of a woman's face with her hand resting across her mouth, cutting off her voice. And to another wooden sculpture I carved with an inscription: "Take seriously my own voice."

Lying in bed, I contemplate what it would mean *not* to bite my tongue. To speak my mind. Despite everything—legal training, assertiveness training, feminism, therapy—I'm still hard-wired to be nice.

Tanya and I are on our way out of town, now that I'm talking again, and we bump into Helen, whose sons are Cooper's age and away at college, too. I dash into the bakery to get bran muffins and chai, and when I return, she's still there, talking to Tanya. She asks how I am, and I pause, thinking about what to tell her.

"Life is complicated," I say. "I have tongue cancer. I've had surgery, and now I have six weeks of radiation to go."

"If it comes back, are they going to cut out your whole tongue? If they do, you can learn sign language with me," she says. "It's really fun!" She's actually *perky* as she says this. She's as clueless as Sally was at the mediation training all those years ago the first time I had cancer.

I'm *so* shocked I can barely take a breath. What I want to say is this: "Are you *crazy*? What kind of response is that?" But the nice girl intervenes and says, "Actually, I'm quite optimistic that the treatment is going to work, so I hadn't thought of that."

Which is true. Having my whole tongue cut out has never even entered my mind. Now I have a new horror for my imagination to gnaw on in the middle of the night.

Julia, age nine, and Margaret, age twelve, knock on my front door. They live across the street from us, and we've known both of them since they were born. Julia is a rowdy tomboy with a face full of purple braces and an A's baseball cap. Margaret is a tall, blond little lady, delicate and proper. It's lovely to have children in the neighborhood now that Cooper is gone.

"Is it Girl Scout cookie time?" I ask as I invite them inside.

"No, we're returning the bowl from the strawberries you brought us."

They help themselves to a seat on the couch as our dog, Mollie, jumps all over them, licking their cheeks and ears.

"Can you get our newspapers on Saturday and Sunday?" they ask.

"Sure, where are you going?"

"To Monterey. We're going to the aquarium. It's our spring break."

We chat about this and that, and then Margaret turns to me, looks at me directly, and asks, "How's your tongue?"

"It's good," I say. "I can talk. It doesn't hurt right now. I feel good."

She smiles, relief apparent.

Like most people with cancer, I can't help but wonder, Why me? One of my doctors asked a long series of questions about smoking and drinking. I admitted that I smoked for two years over forty years ago.

I confessed to drinking wine with dinner. After more questions, he said, "This is bad luck. There's no reason you should have gotten this." Will there be a lesson I can wrest from cancer this time? Last time I jumped out of my lawyer head into my vulnerable heart, at least part of the time; I re-connected to my spirit and my emotions. But to be honest, at the moment, I don't feel very inspired about what I'm going through.

But I *am* moved to simplify a bit, like recognizing how much of what we say doesn't matter during those weeks when I couldn't talk. Unfortunately, simplifying involves a certain amount of grief about what's left behind. Long stretches of time at our little cabin on the Russian River will be over when we sell the property. We can't afford the time or money now that I'm not working. I imagine life without this place of peaceful solitude, where my body relaxes and my mind settles. I'll miss those quiet moments. I'm also giving up my beautiful office on Fourth Street to decrease expenses when I go back to work again. I did some of my best work in this space on the second floor. I'd gaze through the tree branches at life on the street, and when the mediation got difficult, the view gave me perspective: life is so much bigger than the dispute in this room. I'll have to work out of my home office. And gone, for the most part, are most of the hours of simple socializing; when you have cancer, anxiety often fills the room.

Still, I like scaling back, spending less, doing less, reading more, creating space, both physical and mental, resting, doing nothing, devoting more time to creative work like cooking and writing. Books get hauled off, furniture goes to the homeless shelter, things I thought I would never part with fly out the door while I smile. Our friend Mollie gets an oak table that David and I bought in the 1970s, Mary gets a bench, Sarah gets a fountain. With each departure, I feel lighter, less encumbered, less tethered to the material world.

BEHAVING BADLY

In January 1970, just before I turn twenty-one, I arrive at the new Bank of America building in downtown San Francisco for a job interview wearing dangling earrings, no pantyhose, and a very short plaid polyester shift. *After* he hires me, the interviewer hands me the employee manual. The dress code requires women to wear pantyhose every day and skirts or dresses no more than two inches above the knee. Pantyhose are expensive and get runs quite easily, especially on the rough Muni seats. All I own is miniskirts. How will I meet the dress requirements on only $400 per month? For a moment, I wonder why I'm leaving Greyhound with its union pay and no dress code.

But then I remember the appeal of regular hours. I've grown tired of working the swing shift at Greyhound.

I become the receptionist in the employment office on the thirteenth floor of the brand-spanking-new bank headquarters on California Street. It's the tallest building in San Francisco, smooth granite and glass. The elevators whoosh up to the higher floors. Contemporary artwork adorns the walls. Everyone is efficient.

Alone in a fluorescent-lighted, windowless room, I greet job seekers and answer five phone lines that ring constantly. My instructions: Male college grads go to Management Training and other men get an interview. All women, college grads or not, take a typing test.

Outside our climate-controlled building, the noisy '70s rage.

Inside, hushed sterility is the norm. At the bank, you'd never know that American life is changing at a rapid clip.

One day, a large young woman with coffee skin and soft brown eyes walks into my office. "I was here a month ago," she says. "They told me to come back."

I reach for the index cards containing information about people who have already been interviewed. I'm supposed to simply give it to her and send her to the back room to wait for another interview, but something tells me to turn the card over. When I do, I see a note in capital letters: TOO UNATTRACTIVE.

My eyes sting with tears. I look right at her. "You don't want to work here," I say. "It's a horrible place." I jot down the name of an employment agent who likes me and that I talk to almost every day. I give her the list of open positions at the bank and she gives me a heads-up about people she's sending for interviews. "Tell her I sent you. She'll help you find a good job."

The woman thanks me politely and leaves.

When she's gone, I try to gather my emotions, but I'm furious and out of control. I absolutely hate working at the bank. My bosses treat me like I don't have a brain. In fact, they treat everyone, especially women, horribly. Not to mention that the bank funds the war in Vietnam. I take a big breath and walk into the luxurious back office where all the windows are and ask to speak to my boss. I rant. I behave *really* badly. When it's over, I won't remember a single thing except that I quit.

My replacement is a college graduate from Smith who has red hair and wears sweater sets with pearls. I train her for a few days and I'm done.

Fortunately, Greyhound welcomes me back with open arms.

On April 30, a week after my last day at the bank, President Nixon announces that the United States has invaded Cambodia. A national day of protest is announced by the usual array of political organizations. Supporters of the protest are instructed to wear black armbands. I make mine out of an old pair of black tights. My plan is to pick up my last paycheck from the bank and attend the demonstration downtown.

When I stroll onto the bank plaza, a contingent of police is guarding the two hundred-ton black granite sculpture by a Japanese sculptor. Protesters call it "The Banker's Heart." It's been defaced with blood-red paint.

I walk into the lobby donning my black armband. Immediately, police officers appear on each side of me. "What's your business?" they ask gruffly.

"I'm picking up my paycheck," I say, a little fearful. San Francisco cops are known to hate protestors.

"We'll escort you."

They stand with me on the elevator as we float up to the thirteenth floor. At the reception area of the Employment Office, the Smith graduate stares at me, wide-eyed, as if I might be a criminal. She hands me my paycheck. Then the police whisk me back onto the elevator, down through the main lobby, and out the doors to the plaza where the Banker's Heart glistens in the sun, ugly, black, impersonal. I'm free!

EMBRACING THE MASK

I'm lying on a cold, hard metal table in the radiology department at Summit Hospital in Oakland for radiation prep. It's been six weeks since they cut out a chunk of my tongue. The table is narrow, not quite as wide as my body, so I feel like I could fall off. My eyes are covered. Two technicians approach and put a warm, malleable, putty-like substance over my entire face. Then they start shaping it: pat, pat, patting. The hole for my nose is so small that I can barely breathe. My ears are covered, and with the exception of a second small hole, my mouth is completely covered, too. This nightmare is part of the preparation for radiation. The purpose of the mask is to hold my head in place each time I get treatment.

The mask gets tighter and tighter as it dries. At some point, the technicians take it off for a moment and stuff a big wad of soft plastic in my mouth. "Bite," one says. The mask goes back on my head and is then clamped down to the metal table so I can't move. I'm left alone in the cold room.

For forty long minutes I lie on the table, held down by the mask, using all my mental powers to stay calm. Machines click and hum all around me, but I see nothing. I'm trembling, trying not to choke, commanding myself not to start kicking and flailing.

Finally, the two techs return to the room, unclamp my head, and take off the mask. Within seconds, I'm sobbing. The doctor comes to my side with his assistant. They pat me, talking softly, telling me I'll be all right.

My mask and I hang out together five days a week while I get radiated. I arrive at radiology, change into a gown, and lie down on the metal table. I reach up for the mouthpiece, mouth first, like an infant seeking the breast, or a fish rising to the surface to snatch food. I bite down on it, and the mask goes on. Then my head is clamped to the table.

During the third week of radiation, the technicians play "The Buena Vista Social Club," loud Cuban music I adore. For twenty minutes, I'm in Cuba. Dancing. Swirling. Moving in the soft tropical breeze.

"This is *so* much better with music," I say afterward.

"We'll play it for you every day if you want. Some people say it messes with their concentration, so just remind us."

I wonder who in the world needs to concentrate while they're getting radiated.

The next day when I arrive, the music is cranked up; four techs, rather than two, greet me, and the session is over before I know it.

Most days after the radiation, I get baptized, in a fashion. I drag my weary body to the Berkeley Y and spend forty minutes water-walking, emptying my brain, meditating, cooling down. Back and forth through the water, breathing deeply, stretching, turning, churning in the water. I greet the regulars with a smile, but I do not talk.

I flash back to the last time my body seemed perfect. It was the late 1970s. I was around thirty, playing hooky from law school with my study buddy Tom. We were at the gay nude beach on the San Mateo coast, and I was almost the only woman there. It was a shimmering day, sunny, not too windy, springtime, abundant wildflowers. We hiked down to the beach and spontaneously found ourselves running wildly in the surf, naked, young, healthy, tan, beautiful. Running was effortless, more like flying, and we squealed with delight.

When I'm water-walking, I feel my body reaching for health, for life, for joy, for peace. I'm young and hearty again. When I'm finished, I feel renewed, vibrant, alive.

—

My hair starts falling out when I'm in the shower. I see it glistening in the sunshine in the drain with soapsuds and water swirling around it. Then I look at my hands and see big clumps. All the hair below the top of my ears is going, in the line following the radiation as it speeds to my neck and jaw.

I'm crying.

In seconds, Tanya steps into the shower and wraps her arms around me, holding me tight.

By the sixth week of radiation, my taste buds are radiated into complete incompetence. Nothing tastes good. In fact, everything tastes *horrible*, metallic and nasty. What a cruel fate for someone who loves to eat.

I'm told that they "should" begin functioning again several weeks after radiation ends. By my calculation, I've got at least another three weeks of this suffering.

My friend Liz tells me about a friend who also lost her sense of taste during radiation. Six months later at a birthday party, she took a sip of champagne and her taste buds instantly woke up.

"I don't care if you're not drinking, Martina," Liz says. "If your taste buds aren't working by the Fourth of July, I'm coming over with a really good bottle of champagne and we're gonna drink it."

The mask is lifted off by hands I cannot see. It's almost my last radiation treatment. I take out the mouthpiece, breathe deeply, and say, "Guys, you haven't *lived* until you've had a hot flash under the mask while you're being radiated."

The techs laugh.

I stand up from the table and fan myself with my hospital gown.

Eric, one of the techs, quietly says, "Come here. I'll wipe your back."

And, ever so gently, he wipes my bare back dry.

People have been so kind through all this it makes my heart ache. Ann, my close friend since the 1970s, organized Martina's Soup Brigade, and people arrived like clockwork, laden with delicious food. Colleagues who have never even been inside my house made vegetarian soup and left it on the front porch if I was too weak to visit. Susan, another close friend since the '70s, regularly delivered her signature homemade yogurt and applesauce. My friend Arlene brought fluffy blue and white striped socks to keep my feet warm. Bubble bath arrived at the front door. Flowers appeared.

Completing radiation is both an enormous relief and a concern, because now there's nothing to do but wait. I remember how it was the first time I had cancer when Cooper was a baby. Even after twenty years, nobody ever used the word "cured." You don't graduate from cancer: you get treatment, and then you go on living. I suppose I could be cancer-free for another thirty years and live a long and healthy life, or I could die of cancer in six months, or I could beat cancer, and die crossing the street on the way to the Y. All I can do at the moment is live my life day by day and *savor* what's important: intimate moments with family and friends, the yellow roses that just bloomed in my backyard, and the wisteria falling over the front fence, so softly blue.

SHANGRI-LA

A real vacation is what David and I need, and backpacking in the Yolla Bolly Wilderness Area in Northern California is the plan. We've been living together at the commune for eleven months, and David has finally graduated with his master's degree. Meanwhile, Little David dropped out of high school. He was hanging out in the Haight with the hippies, driving us crazy, until he moved in with an ex-girlfriend of his father's with children of her own. It has been an intense year. I welcome having more than a few hours alone with my David.

We drive three hours north on Highway 101, through Marin and Sonoma Counties into Mendocino County. But instead of turning west to the famous town of Mendocino, which hangs on the cliffs overlooking the Pacific, we turn east and drive along a narrow forty-mile, two-lane road that winds along the Eel River until it comes to a spot that looks out over Round Valley. In the middle sits a town called Covelo, population 3,000, a mix of cowboys, Native Americans, farmers, and hippies. We stand by the side of the road, gazing out at the valley encircled by mountains, feeling like we've found Shangri-La.

Hot and exhausted from the twisting road, we're too tired to drive to the trailhead and begin our hike. Instead, we check into the Wagon Wheel Motel downtown. Round Valley enchants us. We see lots of young people my age who live there on small plots of land, gardening, building houses, back-to-the landers who have left the city.

We never make it on our backpacking trip. Instead, we fantasize about living in Covelo and learn about an opening for an English teacher at the high school. David wanders into the school and by the end of our second day in town, he has a job. I visit the elementary school and get hired as a teaching assistant in the educationally handicapped class. On the third day, we rent a little house in the middle of the valley, surrounded by open fields and farms, looking out at the hills with no road in sight.

Our commune in San Francisco is at the end of our one-year commitment and everyone is ready to move on. We amicably give up the house. David and I adopt a dog named Dylan, rent a U-Haul, and head north to start over in Covelo.

On my first day in my new job at the elementary school, I'm assigned five first-graders for the morning. Each has learning issues. LeAnne, one of the students in my group, immediately asks, "Mrs. Patton, what church did you go to yesterday?"

Oh, my God! How am I supposed to answer that? And for that matter, who is Mrs. Patton?

It's not like I haven't had a lot of names in my life. My birth name was Ellen Martin Reaves. Martin was my maternal grandmother's maiden name. I think my parents expected to call me Ellen, but when my father saw me, he called me Marti. I remained Marti Reaves until sixth grade when I decided to have a girl's name for a year and called myself Ellen. I reverted to Marti the next year. I'll finally adopt the name Martina years later, when David and I move to Mexico for the summer and I feminize Martin to Martina. The new name sticks. But now, in 1971, to suddenly become a Mrs. with a last name I've never used is shocking.

We'd pretended to be married when we got our jobs, fearful that living together would be considered a sin in this conservative territory. But the truth is that marriage is something we'd *never* thought about.

At this particular moment I have to decide how to respond to Leann about church.

"We just moved here and we haven't figured out where to go yet," I say.

"We go to the Church of God," LeAnne says. The kids then have a long conversation about which churches their families attend. There is no question about *whether* they attend church, only which one. I know better than to tell them I'm a lapsed Unitarian.

That night, we realize we need to get married to keep our jobs. Faking it is just too risky. We plan quickly, and on October 2 we pile into our car and drive to San Francisco for our wedding. Richard, my gay co-worker from Greyhound, hosts the event at his garden cottage on Ord Court just above Castro Street.

The wedding is a scene.

Picture the bride, twenty-one, with the flu, in a peasant dress that her mother purchased in Mexico the week before the wedding. Barefoot. The groom is nineteen years older, with long hair, in a gray jacket with a velvet collar that makes him look like an over-aged British rocker. Richard, the host, wears a red-white-and-blue satin shirt open to the waist, exposing his voluminous roly-poly stomach, his boyfriend at his side. Our friends are a mixture of teachers, artists, hippies, students, and Muni employees. My parents, various relatives, and Navy colleagues are dressed appropriately for an old-fashioned wedding. Both of my brothers, hair down to their shoulders, are squeezed into jackets that my parents insisted they wear. David's friend, Jim, another lapsed Episcopal priest, officiates in an oversized white Mexican shirt.

The morning starts out foggy, but by the time of the wedding it's a wonderful, clear, sunny, warm day, typical of October in San Francisco. There's lots of champagne, delicious food, and nobody leaves early, except my father, who gets tipsy on champagne and returns to the hotel.

David and I spend our wedding night at The Golden Hinde Boatel in Inverness on the coast north of San Francisco. Unfortunately, in all the commotion, I leave my clothing, except for the blue jeans and T-shirt I'm wearing, in a closet at the Beck Motor Inn on Market Street in San Francisco. At the only store in Inverness, I buy an ugly plaid dress, and we eat a sumptuous dinner at Manka's, where wealthy, properly dressed folks eye us warily. Finally, we collapse into a heap in our room overlooking Tomales Bay, too exhausted for anything resembling romance.

By Monday morning, I'm legally Martin Reaves Patton and we're back in our Covelo classrooms, acting as if we've had another quiet country weekend.

During the school year, we learn that David needs a teaching credential to continue with his job. His provisional credential lasts for one year only. And I discover that I want to finish college. I want to be taken seriously; I sense that my opinion is dismissed in favor of David's because I don't have a degree. It hasn't dawned on me that I'm being dismissed because I'm young and female; feminism isn't even a word in my vocabulary yet. For the moment, I just want to learn.

When school ends in June, we load up a U-Haul and head north with Trippy, the mellow dog we traded for Dylan so Dylan could live on a ranch instead of in town. We leave Shangri-La for Ashland, Oregon, where David can quickly get his credential and I can study.

I thrive at Southern Oregon College. I take painting, sculpture, psychology, sociology, and independent studies classes I design myself. Rather than returning to Covelo for the next school year, David gets a job at the Youth Project and I finish college. I attend classes year-round and fifteen months later, I'm a graduate.

At this point, we notice teaching jobs advertised in the Virgin Islands. And they need both of us, David for high school English and me for kindergarten. David checks a map and sees that St. Thomas is near Puerto Rico. He thinks he'll be able to use his degree in Teaching English as a Foreign Language because there will be Puerto Ricans there. On a whim, we apply and are hired at the last minute in August, just before school starts in September.

The number of Puerto Ricans we find on St. Thomas: none.

St. Thomas teems with life: kids yelling, dogs barking, horns tooting, music blasting, parents yelling, mosquitoes buzzing, mice skittering, cockroaches crunching, lizards slithering, everyone laughing, laughing, laughing. There isn't a quiet spot on the island.

David and I briefly live in the concrete basement apartment of some expats in Red Hook on the other side of the island from the main town, Charlotte Amalie, while we look for a place to rent. A one-bedroom, plywood shack with a tin roof at the end of a dirt road is all we can afford on our teachers' salaries. No breezy waterfront condo for us. Rainwater collects from the rooftop and runs down under the house into a cistern, where it is held until it is pumped back up into the house for our use. When we first arrive, nobody tells us we need to boil the water before drinking it, and we both get deathly ill.

David teaches at the high school in Charlotte Amalie, the main city that overlooks the harbor. I'm stuck in Madison School, a little country school in the middle of the island where there is not one speck of breeze from the sea. It's so crowded that we have double sessions; my kindergarten class runs from 12:30 to 5:30 with a single fifteen-minute break.

Early every morning, David takes our only car, a VW bug, and drives to town to get to work at 8 a.m. Later, I shower, dress for work, and walk down the dirt road from our house to catch the school bus to work. By the time I reach the bus stop, I'm always drenched with sweat. The bus bounces along the narrow winding roads to school and disgorges chattering little black kids and one drooping white teacher.

My classroom is so tiny that the only things that fit into it are one teacher's desk and the four small tables where the children sit in plastic chairs. Louvered windows stretch along two walls. At each end of the room are doors to the outside and a minuscule, stinky bathroom shoots off one end next to the entry door. That is it.

"I'm Mrs. Patton," I say, the first day of school. I look at the squirming kids at their tables and wonder how these little beings will be able to sit in those chairs for five hours.

"Missus Pat-on, you talk funny," Catharine (pronounced Katarin) says with a lilt. Tiny, wiry, deep black, exuberant, funny, she is always laughing, especially at me.

Fortunately I have Vernice, newly arrived on St. Thomas from one of the British Virgin Islands, who translates for the first month of school. She is the only child in my class that I can understand. Vernice looks at me with her green eyes and café au lait skin, astonished that I can't understand what the other children are saying. Then she carefully repeats their words in her dialect until I understand.

My principal is an old-fashioned school-marm type. She wears her hair pulled up into a bun, sensible shoes, and long flowered dresses belted at the waist. Ancient and strict, she's reminiscent of my sour Southern aunt, except she's black and speaks in a thick dialect.

The first week of school, in the middle of the hottest part of the afternoon, I take the kids outside for a movement exercise I learned in the educationally handicapped class in Covelo. They line up behind me and then copy my movements as we snake around the dusty schoolyard.

After school, the principal's assistant tells me that the principal wants to talk to me. "You can't take the children outside in the middle of the afternoon," she says, without looking up from her paperwork. "What if their parents came by and saw you out there? They would think the children weren't learning." I explain that they were learning by moving. She is unmoved, completely uninterested in new ideas, especially mine.

David doesn't fare any better. He is supposed to teach traditional English classes and have the students read the "classics," meaning British and early American authors. Most of the kids are completely bored and barely participate.

He decides to approach things in a different way, as if he were teaching standard English as a second language. He finds Caribbean writers whose books relate to the lives of his students. The dialogue is in their dialect. When he gives these books to the kids, they gobble them up, the discussions are interesting, they're excited to write and read. He talks to them about language, about dialect, about standard American English, and about why they might want to learn it because of the doors it could open for them.

It isn't long before the chair of his department calls him into her office. Speaking to him in dialect, she says, "We don't speak in dialect here. What are you talking about? Only Communists talk like you." The C word is laden, since the golf course shootings by avowed radicals on St. Croix had just taken place. She directly orders David to teach the standard curriculum: Byron, Keats, Shelley, Thoreau, Emerson.

Being white on an island that is ninety percent black is complicated, if not strange. The only other white people besides teachers are sailing bums, the wealthy owners of beach-side properties, and a handful of shop owners. Most of the whites are visitors, either the sun-baskers in condos on the beaches or the ubiquitous, mostly Southern tourists who stream off cruise ships for four hours of duty-free shopping in Charlotte Amalie and then retreat to their pristine ships with piles of bags filled with French perfume, silk scarves, and designer clothes. It is understandable that locals don't have high regard for white people, but it still feels horrible to be treated like one of those loud, rude, inconsiderate tourists. Walking into a store and having the shopkeeper attend to anyone black and ignore me while I patiently wait is hard to take.

After a while I devise a strategy: The first time I walk through the door of any new store, no matter what I need, I talk about Madison School. I want the shopkeeper to know I'm local, not a rich tourist. The mere mention of Madison School initiates animated conversation about the shopkeeper's cousin or niece or nephew who attends, and then we are friends.

David and I are poor, really poor, with just enough money to buy Kentucky Fried chicken for dinner once a week. Twice a month, if we're careful, we can afford a restaurant that caters to locals. We dress in our finest and sit in lounge chairs while the breeze blows in from the sea. We eat fish and drink piña coladas and pretend we're living the good life. But the truth is that at the end of each month, there isn't a penny left in our checking account until our next paychecks arrive.

David gets home from school every day at 3:30. I arrive at home by bus at 6. We pile into our VW and drive to a secret beach near our house that is always empty at that hour. We sink into the cool, salty, buoyant water and wash away the day, facing the brilliant orange sky as the sun sets. Then we come home, eat, and fall onto our foam mattress on the floor to sleep, naked and always, always hot and sweating.

CELEBRATE

The unimaginable happens in June 2008: the California Supreme Court says that same-sex couples can get married! I'm in the midst of sending an email to my so-called "cancer list," and instead of just giving them details about my cracked, snakeskin neck and my radiated taste buds and telling them my radiation is complete, I can write about something besides cancer.

"And now," I write, "Tanya and I can get married after twenty-seven-plus years together. Tanya 'proposed' yesterday. I told her to get on her knees. She said, 'Not until you finish vacuuming the kitchen floor.'"

To be totally honest, calling it twenty-seven-plus years is a bit misleading, given our early years of Lesbian High Drama of splitting up and getting back together. Over the years, whenever anyone asked us how long we'd been together, we often gave different answers. I gave the date we finally got back together and stayed together and Tanya gave the date we first realized we were, as they say, "more than friends." Finally, we agreed to use Tanya's date because we both know that we'd needed the LHD years to realize what we meant to each other. We now count from December 6, 1980.

Completing radiation and planning a wedding would have been plenty to celebrate, but there's more: Cooper's graduation from college. He's returned from his semester in Costa Rica and is back at Cornell College in Iowa. Tanya and I fly to Chicago and hop onto a tiny plane that takes us to Cedar Rapids, Iowa. I look down at a landscape of orderly fields with occasional splashes of trees and meandering creeks and rivers. Cooper picks us up at the airport and drives us through the abundant green landscape to our motel on the outskirts of pristine Mount Vernon, Iowa.

After we unload, we stretch out on the beds. Cooper watches me intently, searching my face for clues. I can see him wondering if I'm okay. In truth, I probably look better than the last time I saw him; I'm thinner, more rested, and less stressed, at least in some ways.

The weekend is a flurry of activities. Meeting professors, classmates, and other families. Celebratory meals. The ceremony. Packing his car for his drive back to California with a friend. When Tanya and I fly home on Sunday, I'm exhausted and happy.

Now we can focus on the wedding.

In July, I have a routine PET scan, my first since completing radiation, and after several days, the results come in: Everything is fine with my tongue, my mouth, and everything else in my body, but there's one lymph node in my neck that's problematic. It will have to be removed. The cancer isn't gone. . .

This news is so shocking it feels almost like a third diagnosis of cancer. I'd begun to feel like myself again and even started to work part-time, all the while ignoring my deep fear about that tiny lymph node that had been sore and puffy throughout radiation.

We head into another surgery. Another recovery. Another round of telling my clients I can't work.

PARADISE LOST

On the last day of school in St. Thomas, just after my students graduate from my kindergarten class, Mr. Amey, one of the fathers, looks at me and says, "Please come back next year."

"Don't worry," I say. "I'm coming back." And I truly mean it.

He smiles. "So many don't come back," he says with a wistful look on his face. He's referring to all the mainlanders who teach a year or two and then move on.

The following week, David and I get a sitter for our house and Trippy the dog and head to Mexico for two months to study Spanish. We live in a small village outside Oaxaca. Nobody owns a car; the bus goes into Oaxaca in the morning and returns in the afternoon.

I change my name to Martina to feminize Martin. It's the first time I love my name.

We live with a family of potters and sleep in their storage shed, helping Doña Rebeca cook beans and make tortillas on a daily basis. This involves sifting the beans to remove pebbles and removing the corn kernels from dried cornhusks so they can be ground up for tortillas. David accompanies Don Francisco with the burro to mine clay and gather firewood for cooking and firing the pottery. Each night, after a long day of working to provide for the family, Doña Rebeca begins her paid work building huge pots that are used to hold water. Each family in the village has a specialty.

Our plan is to practice Spanish while we live with our family and then spend a few weeks in California before returning to St. Thomas for the 1973–74 school year.

It isn't until we get to the Bay Area and are enveloped into the arms of friends that returning to St. Thomas begins to seem impossible. Impossible despite the fact that the children were the most amazing human beings I've ever encountered. They vibrated joy. Black faces, brown faces, coffee and cream faces, smiling, always smiling, fully inhabiting their bodies, wiggly, giggly, effervescent.

Me, the white teacher from California who thought I knew a lot, but really knew next to nothing about teaching, next to nothing about the Virgin Islands, next to nothing about much of anything, really. Freshly graduated from college, I was on another adventure with David—both of us from Navy families, both infected with wanderlust.

Back in California, I remember how homesick I was all year. Despite spending our lives moving, first in our Navy families and thereafter by choice, neither of us adjusted well. Usually a person with many friends, I had none in the Virgin Islands.

We got through the year because of the delicious sweetness of the kids, the desire to do good work, and the beaches. But it was a really hard year. Though we originally intended to go back, in a selfish, desperate move, we decide not to return. I feel guilty, thinking of earnest Mr. Amey.

I have to slink back to the Virgin Islands alone to get our dog and our things while David looks for work in California. Stuffing two huge suitcases with what we need immediately, I pack our remaining belongings into boxes to ship home and make arrangements to fly Trippy to SFO. All the while, I hope I don't run into any parents from last year's class. Fortunately, I see nobody I know.

David returns to Round Valley and lands a job as director of the

Youth Project with what was then called the Indian Tribal Council in Covelo. He writes grants to obtain funding for projects in the valley that will help the native community. I become one of two kindergarten teachers in the elementary school where I'd previously worked as an aide.

We rent a little cabin on the Eel River, about thirty minutes from town. After the intimacy of the Virgin Islands, where it was impossible to find solitude, we love the isolation, the silence, the raging water, the huge boulders that line the banks of the river between our cabin and the river.

We awaken early each morning. David builds a fire, we do yoga, and then we bathe. Our cabin has a stone fireplace and no hot water, so we heat icy-cold well water in a big pot on the propane stove, soap up, and dribble warm water down our bodies to rinse off in front of the fire.

In the spring, Patty Hearst is kidnapped by a radical group called the Symbionese Liberation Army. The Hearsts, a San Francisco newspaper family, provide food for the poor as part of a deal to try to get Patty back. David decides to apply for some of the food for members of the tribe he is working for, most of whom are grindingly poor. But when he tells his boss about the plan, his boss says, "We don't want blood money. Don't take the food."

Thinking that food for the hungry is more important than his boss's principles, David arranges for the food to be donated to the tribe through another youth project so that it doesn't come directly from the Hearst Corporation. Cheese, flour, grains, and peanut butter arrive in pickup trucks and are distributed to grateful tribal members. But David's boss figures out the origin of the food and things devolve quickly. David is immediately fired. My principal, who has promised me a job the next school year, says, "You're too controversial to teach here."

—

Run out of Shangri-La, we move fifty miles away to Ukiah, the county seat of Mendocino County, where David becomes director of the Mendocino County Youth Project and I work at the family planning clinic, providing information about birth control, STDs, and abortions. It's 1974, the time of consciousness raising, rising feminism, rebellion, and alternative lifestyles. It's during this time that I finally find my real name: Martina Ellen Reaves. I take back my own last name and get a credit card in my name instead of David's, wresting my identity from being Mrs. Patton.

After living in town a year, we buy fifty acres in the hills outside town down a long dirt road. Our home is an old Airstream trailer with a huge screened-in porch, a woodstove, propane lamps, no electricity, and no running water. We live off the grid. Each weekend, we drive our pickup to a waterfall at the lowest point on our property. There, we fill a metal drum with water, haul it back to our trailer, and pump the water to a holding tank up the hill that gravity-feeds it to our sink and shower.

Mendocino County is loaded with hippies like us who live in the country and barely scrape by.

CRAZY-MAKING DAYS

There's something crazy-making about planning a wedding while scheduling a surgery for cancer, but we do it anyway. We're worried—as it later turns out, correctly—that our right to marry won't last long. Within months of that initial June 2008 celebration, same-sex marriage becomes illegal again. Our invitations go out barely a month before the wedding date, with a note that says we've waited for my surgeon to say I could dance at our wedding. "Dress as you please," the invitation continues. "Tanya will be in cowgirl boots and jeans. Martina will be dressed more appropriately, so there's a full range of possibilities before you. Jeans and boots or black tie, you choose. Bring your dancing shoes; we have an all-girl band."

"You know, people die from that," my brother Warren announces to my mother and Tanya. It's August, the day after my neck surgery, just a few weeks before the wedding. My blood pressure is 80/40. I have a six-inch slice in the side of my neck where the surgeon removed multiple lymph nodes, including the one that we know the tongue cancer had quietly sneaked into. I'm in intensive care, happily loaded on pain medication, gazing at Tanya, Warren, and my mother at the foot of my bed.

Warren, a nurse, launches into a lecture on the four ways you can die when your blood pressure is this low. Space out, I say to myself, and I float away. When I come back, Tanya looks horrified. My mother nods, impressed with Warren's knowledge.

The next day, my mother and brother appear just as my surgeon arrives.

"Good morning," the doctor smiles, altogether cordial as he shakes hands with my mother and brother and nods at Tanya. He leans over me in the bed and gently removes the bandage.

"Can I have a mirror?" I say. "I want to see what it looks like."

A long row of huge staples stares back at me from the side of my neck. I look like a horror ready for Halloween. The surgeon inspects closely, touches tenderly, and says, "Beautiful."

Coming out of the end of the incision is a small tube that drains fluid as it accumulates. "I'm going to take the drain out now," my surgeon says.

And at that very moment, my mother and brother start pummeling him with questions. "How was the surgery?" "When will we get the pathology report?" "How long will it take to heal?"

The doctor's head bounces back and forth like a ping pong ball. He looks at the work he's trying to do. He turns to make eye contact with them. He snips the stitch that's holding the drain to my neck. Looks at them to answer a question. Comes back to me to snip another stitch.

Tanya gently puts her hand on my mother's lap and says quietly but firmly, "Judy, can you and Warren please stop asking questions so that he can get that thing out of her neck?" Momentary silence.

"Ready?" the doctor says. Floop. The six-inch tube emerges from the end of the incision, like a snake shedding its skin. A sudden flash of pain, and it's over.

The doctor had told me to expect five nights in the hospital.

In the middle of the first night, I get up to walk the halls, arm in arm with Tanya. We drag my body down the fluorescent halls, past open doorways with comatose patients, gathering dust balls on my socks. It seems wrong that there are dust balls in the hospital, but I ignore them and breathe deeply. I stretch. I'll do anything to get myself out of here.

I'm such a good patient that I'm home after only two nights. The initial pathology report confirms that the first two nodes were cancerous. We wait to hear about the approximately forty other nodes that were removed.

I now know how to do recuperation. Lots of reading: *New Yorkers* and a pile of good books. Frequent naps. Short walks with the dog. The gash in my neck is rather frightening, so I mostly hibernate until the staples come out. Eight days after surgery, my surgeon snips them off, and I'm left with my six-inch battle scar.

"What about the pathology report?" I ask.

The surgeon shuffles through the papers in the file. "This can't be the final pathology report. It's just not here yet. I'll call you when it comes in."

He seems utterly oblivious to the anxiety created by the long wait.

"This space is beautiful," I say to Barbara, who owns the Montclair Women's Cultural Arts Center. It glows. Luscious paintings hang on maroon walls. It's steeped with history. Modern but timeless. Voluptuous flower arrangements. "I'm so glad we're having our wedding here."

Tanya tastes two red wines, three white wines, two champagnes, and makes her choices. I haven't had alcohol since January, when I was first diagnosed. It's against the doctor's orders. Besides, with my radiated taste buds, it would taste bitter and sour.

"What color tablecloths?"

We choose burgundy and plum.

"Do you want all the candles lit?"

Of course.

We run through the timing of the afternoon, and that's that.

In the afternoon we head off to see the radiologist for a routine check-up, and it occurs to me to ask him about the pathology report, since we still haven't heard from the surgeon. I show him the initial pathology report that was done in the middle of surgery, the one that showed cancer in the first two nodes that were removed. I tell him we're waiting for the final report.

The radiologist calls Pathology. He looks at us, bewildered, and says that Pathology says they have no other specimens to analyze.

Tanya and I go into detective mode. I harass my doctor's office for days until he produces a written surgery report, something that should have been created at the time of the surgery. I fax it to Pathology and call the pathologist to ask her to review the report to see whether the pathology report we have matches up with it.

To her credit, she actually calls me back and says that they don't match up, that she's going to conduct an "investigation."

And it's then that I know with certainty that my tissue is long gone. That we'll never find out whether there were more cancerous nodes in my neck.

Two days later, she calls me to say she has searched the entire lab, and that no other samples from my surgery were ever logged in to Pathology.

"How often does this happen?" I ask her.

"Almost never," she says.

Inside, I rage at my doctor, who doesn't call me back, despite the numerous messages I've left him.

"I need dancing shoes for the wedding," I say to Tanya. "Shoes that are pretty, not the ones I use in dance class." After a thorough search of Berkeley and Oakland, we realize we might need to have leather put on the bottom of shoes I already own, to make them slide on the dance floor.

We practice our West Coast swing routine to "Sweet Inspiration," trying to perfect our moves. Half the time we forget the order of our choreography and end up laughing.

"I believe in learning from experience," the oncologist says. "You have two lymph nodes that survived the radiation. They're gone. But there may be more small cancer cells left. I strongly recommend three months of chemotherapy."

I want to throw up.

"What kind of chemotherapy? More powerful than the chemo I had in 1986 for the lymphoma?"

"Yes."

His blue eyes are piercing. He doesn't blink. The man could sell anything to anybody. He wants to start chemo the *day after the wedding!*

"I'm not doing anything without a second opinion at this point," I say. "I have an appointment at UCSF."

"For this type of cancer, I'd go to Stanford, not UCSF."

"If I call Stanford now, I won't get in for six weeks."

"We'll get you in before that."

Which is how I find myself at the Stanford Comprehensive Cancer Center in early September, a few days before our September 14 wedding. Fifteen doctors from the Tumor Board parade through my room. They cram their fingers down my throat. They feel my neck, press fingers into my scar, put tubes down my nose, mumbling all the time to each other.

"Wouldn't have done the radiation."

"Why a second opinion now?"

"Tissue looks good."

"Why not a full neck resection, rather than this partial?" (Translation: Why did my surgeon only cut out *some* of the neck, rather than all of it?)

Tanya and I are dismissed and told to return at 11:45 a.m. for the verdict.

Nervous, we keep ourselves occupied by searching for wedding shoes at Nordstrom.

When we reconvene, the chief of the head and neck oncology department says, "I can't give you a second opinion without talking to your surgeon." This is especially true because of the missing biopsy results. "But I can tell you this: The only question is whether to do the full neck resection. We don't recommend chemotherapy."

"How many doctors were in the room?"

"About fifteen."

"Did *any* of them recommend chemotherapy?"

"No. Not one. Unfortunately, chemotherapy does not cure head and neck cancers. There's no reason for you to have chemo now. We have no reason to think you have cancer at all."

Tanya and I are euphoric. Surgery I can handle. But not three more months of chemo and its aftermath.

The marriage clerk's waiting room is filled with people, all kinds of people, and electric with energy. There's an African American family: a bride dressed in white, carrying a corsage, a groom, kids, and old folks, all dressed in their finest. There's a young couple in power suits, hair coiffed, nails perfect, looking important with their leather briefcases. They can barely look at the rest of us in the room, and you can tell, just by looking at them, that they'll spend more than $100,000 on their wedding. There's Tanya and me, two middle-aged (or old, depending upon your perspective) lesbians in blue jeans and T-shirts. We're all applying for marriage licenses.

Our number is finally called.

"We have a problem," I say. "We need my friend to be deputized to perform the wedding. I went on line and found out that you wanted us to submit paperwork three weeks ago. I'm hoping you can help us. I was in the hospital three weeks ago." I turn my head and show her my inflamed, six-inch scar. "I couldn't do this until now."

She looks at us and shakes her head. "They won't do it," she says. Then she adds, "But I'll call up there and see what I can do." She leaves her desk and phones from the back of the room. I can't hear what she's saying, but when she returns, she's smiling. We get our license and approval for Ann to perform the ceremony.

Ann and I meet at a salon to have manicures and pedicures, a pre-wedding treat. There's something vaguely uncomfortable to me about the whole process. The mostly Asian women wait on us, hand and foot. The super-feminine atmosphere makes me feel like an impostor, an intruder who doesn't belong.

Ann announces that I'm getting married, which is met with oooohs and ahhhhs. I wonder what they would think if they knew I'm marrying a woman. But slowly, my body relaxes into the pillows surrounding me; my feet sink into the warm, sudsy water. I could get used to this, I think.

An elegant woman walks into the room from the back of the salon. She moves like a model, smoothly slinking toward me. Her hair is very short, spiky blond with dark roots. Plain gold jewelry adorns her wrists and neck. She looks like a Thai dancer.

She moves to a stool by me and says in a very deep voice that she's going to do my manicure. The only thing that's masculine about her is her voice.

A few moments later, she calls across the room to an older, African American woman, telling her what treatment she will want the next time she comes. The woman leaves. "She's a very nice woman," she says, turning back to me. "She comes every week, but she's sad. She and her partner got married in June, and her partner died two months later. They were together over thirty years."

I tell her, then, that I'm marrying my partner of twenty-eight years. She says, "Are you going to have children?"

I almost laugh out loud. She can't possibly think I can still have children! "We already have a child," I say. "He's twenty-two now."

"I'm twenty-two, too," she says.

An hour later, I'm fluffed, massaged, beautified, and relaxed.

A few days before the wedding, I write my vows, which I've been thinking about for over a month:

"What kind of vow can I make to you? You moved into my heart twenty-eight years ago and set up housekeeping. At first, I tried to evict you. Then, I slowly moved in with you. You've been rumbling around down there, remodeling, making art, laughing, chattering to me all this time with your blue eyes twinkling. I feel so blessed to have found you. How improbable our connection was, and how wonderful it's been.

We've already done for richer or poorer, for better or worse, in sickness and in health. You've been there, unflinching, through wonderful times and horrible times, and at each step, you fill up more space in my heart, even when I thought there was no more room to expand.

So, I promise to do all I can to keep my heart open.

I promise to always make room for fun.

I promise, when I'm feeling invisible, furious, and out of control, to remember that at least eighty percent of it is not about you at all.

I promise to dance as much as possible.

I promise to support you to do the things that are important to you.

I promise to be as honest as I can with you.

And most of all, I promise to love you with every fiber of my being."

Our wedding is the only thing in my life that ever went without a hitch. It was perfect, full of laughter, tears, hugs, kisses, music, dancing, food, and drink. More love in one room than I could have imagined.

It was actually *better* than my fantasies.

UKIAH LIFE

By the mid-'70s, Mendocino County is filled with people fleeing urban areas in search of a quieter life in the country. For the first time in my life, I become part of a community. After working at the family planning clinic, I get a job at the Ukiah Community Center. We work on a Simple Living Workshop that involves gardening techniques, home building, water systems, back-to-the land technology. I work with a social worker from the Department of Social Services to create a single-mothers' support group for women on welfare who are trying to build new lives for themselves and their children. On behalf of the Mendocino County Schools, I research and publish a booklet of all the human services available in the county.

From the first Simple Living Workshop, women's consciousness-raising groups emerge. I meet with my group weekly. Mendocino County Women Against Rape evolves and later morphs into a support group for victims of domestic violence, since the need is so great.

After a year, the temporary funding for my job ends. What next? Reluctant to try public school teaching again, I land a part-time job at the Ukiah daycare center. On my first day, the director introduces me to Diane, my assistant. We're assigned the three-year-olds.

Diane is immediately fascinating to me. She's a black albino—African American features with pale skin, yellow hair, and light blue eyes. Raised in Oakland, she had two kids when she was very young and then joined Peoples Temple in the early '70s. She's a city girl, living in the country for the first time.

Peoples Temple, a church with lefty politics and a commitment to social action, is the only multi-racial religious group I've ever encountered. Its members are political, articulate, and vibrant, with intelligent, thoughtful things to say, always challenging the status quo on behalf of the poor.

At the family planning clinic during my first job in Ukiah I had two colleagues from the temple who were smart, hard-working, and politically active. The woman I collaborated with to start the single-mothers' group during my job at the community center was also a member of the temple. At every community meeting, members of the temple voice progressive, smart suggestions. Folks from the temple are respected all over the county.

That Diane is a member is just another positive thing about her. We work together seamlessly. If I'm doing circle time and one of the kids is acting out, she's right there with that kid so that there's no disruption to the group. If things are smooth, she's there outside the circle, smiling and glowing, singing along. "If you're happy and you know it, clap your hands." Or, "I like Sammy, there's no doubt about it, I like Sammy, there's no doubt about it."

We have snippets of conversation over the heads of the kids as they play and work and yell and fight. "What music should we put on now?" I ask.

"Holly Near," she says.

"What'd you do last weekend?"

"Went to a rally in San Francisco," she says.

"Want a ride?" I ask her after work one day when I see her walking from our center. She nods and climbs into my Mustang. "Where to?"

She directs me to her house. "Where are your kids?" I ask.

"They live in another house with kids their age. Temple kids don't live with their parents." I'm a bit surprised, at first, since her kids are so young, perhaps under twelve. But then, she mentions kibbutzim in Israel, where children live in dorms together. She says their kids' houses are modeled after them.

"Do you get to see them?"

"Regularly," she says. "It's better this way. They get raised by lots of caring adults."

As time goes by, I begin to notice aspects of the temple that seem odd. All the blinds at Diane's house are drawn, even on a sunny day. Her housemates are other People's Temple folks. When I drop her off, I usually see someone peeking out from the curtain of her living room like they're spying on us. Every time we arrive, she gets nervous and fidgety and quickly gets out of the car.

"What's this about?" I finally ask her.

"We're not supposed to spend a lot of time with people who aren't in the temple," she says.

"Why?"

"Because there's so much we're trying to do to make the world a better place that a friendship with someone outside the temple is seen as taking away our focus." It almost feels like a rehearsed response.

I respect the fervor, but the spying seems a bit overzealous.

Almost every Monday morning she comes to work exhausted. "We went to L.A. for the weekend," she often says, "and I didn't get more than a few hours' sleep."

"What do you do there?"

"We meet with the temple members in LA and do political work—leafleting, rallies, stuff like that."

"Where do you sleep?"

"On the bus or at the church."

I ask her more about the temple. She tells me that men and women are treated equally and that as a community they have struggled with and succeeded in dealing with classism and racism. College-educated professionals work side-by-side with folks who never graduated from high school.

We begin to spend more and more time together after work. We have tea. We chat on the playground when the afternoon staff is on duty. We talk about the kids in our class. I worry about one of them, whose mother is dysfunctional. Her son comes to school hungry, wearing filthy clothes, and smelling horrible. I bathe him in the utility closet and put clean clothes on him so that the other kids won't make fun of him. I'm distraught about how he's living, ready to take him home with me.

"There's nothing more you can do," she says. "It's not at a level where they'd take him from his mother's care."

"Why not? What he's going through is horrible," I say.

"Trust me," she says. "The welfare department doesn't do much unless there's obvious violence."

One Friday after work she tells me that Peoples Temple is moving the rest of their members back to the City.

This feels vague to me so I look right at her. "Does that mean you're going to leave?"

"Probably." She looks away.

I'm stunned.

"What will you do there?"

"There's an antique store on Divisadero Street that's run by members of the temple. I'm going to work there."

I say nothing, show nothing. I feel numb.

But over the weekend I erupt. Every time I think about her leaving, I cry. No matter where I am or whom I'm with, tears flow. This emotion makes no sense to me. I've moved all my life, left close friends behind, left boyfriends behind. By the time I was eighteen, I'd lived in at least fourteen different places all over the world. With David, I've lived in ten more. I've never felt this way before.

I go to see my close friend Maggie from my consciousness-raising group. I drive ten miles down the winding road from our land into Ukiah, north on the Highway 101 freeway, and then east to Potter Valley to visit her. I need to talk. We sit on her big, overstuffed couch by the wood stove, drinking tea. I'm crying, shaky, and confused. We talk, but I still can't figure out what's going on with me.

I go home, retracing my drive, down the little dirt road off the Boonville Grade to our cabin. David and I sit on our couch in front of our fire. "What's going on?" he asks.

"I don't understand all this feeling," I say. "I'm so sad about Diane moving. I can't imagine going to work without her. I feel connected to her, like she understands me. When she's in the City, I'll never see her. She'll be busy with the temple, in L.A. on the weekends." I'm in tears.

He listens intently as I ramble. Finally, he says, "I think you're in love with her."

His words feel like an electric jolt. Oh my God, I think. That's what this is. He's right. I just didn't have any frame of reference for it.

Monday at work, Diane and I are setting things up in our classroom. Water colors. Blocks. Books. "I cried all weekend about your leaving," I finally say. "I think I love you. I have no idea what this means. But that's what it feels like."

Her eyes widen and she looks terrified. "We can't do this. You're married. And I can't be with someone outside the temple."

Just then, thankfully, parents and kids arrive, and I go on automatic to get through the day. Snack time. Circle time. Lunch. Naps. Meeting with parents. Home.

The next few weeks are a blur. We work. We talk. "I'm not going to be with you," she says emphatically. "It just isn't possible. You're wonderful, but we aren't going to do this." I don't argue with her. I haven't a clue what I want anyway. I just long for her.

The day before she's leaving for the City, she comes with me out to our land for a few hours after work. She wants to see where I live. It's the first time that we've done anything other than talk after work, have a cup of coffee or tea, or ride together in the car to her house. She lets it slip that she's gotten in trouble with the temple for spending time with me, although she doesn't explain what that means.

It's a sunny, warm spring day, and we walk together arm in arm along the dirt road that passes through our land. I show her all the things we've done—the water system, the daffodils, the garden, the yurt where my brother Whit lives farther down the road. I can feel her skin next to mine as we move. We fit together perfectly, like twins. It feels comfortable.

The next day when she leaves work for the last time, she tells me not to look her up in San Francisco, that she won't be able to spend time with me and keep her commitments to the temple. She hugs me, and then she's gone.

We never even kissed.

During the next year, when I'm in the city to visit friends, I drive along Divisadero past the antique store where I think she works. I crane my neck, drive slowly, and hope to get a glimpse, but I never do. Over time, I stop thinking about her and life with David returns to its equilibrium. In a sense, I'm relieved. I don't like having my boat rocked and being overwhelmed with feeling.

By November 1978, it's been over a year since Diane left Ukiah and I haven't heard a word. But I know from the news that most members of the temple have moved to Jonestown in Guyana. Congressman Leo

Ryan flies there to investigate whether members of Peoples Temple are being kept in Jonestown against their will. Former members are interviewed. The temple, previously the darling of left-wing San Francisco politicians, is now described in the media as a "cult." People begin to distance themselves.

It's Thanksgiving. The news arrives slowly, in bits and pieces. Leo Ryan has been killed at the airstrip as he was leaving Jonestown. There's been a mass suicide. Some people are still alive in the jungle. Names of the dead dribble out. Diane's name isn't among them. The woman I did the single-mothers' group with has been a spokesperson for the Temple in the capital city in Guyana. The news says that upon hearing of the suicides at Jonestown, she slit her children's throats and killed herself. The horror is simply unimaginable.

Photos of the dead finally arrive. They lie face down, rotting in the jungle heat. I scan their backs to see if I can recognize Diane, but I can't tell a thing.

My parents are up from San Diego for Thanksgiving. It's gray, cold, and damp on our land in Ukiah. I dream that Diane has escaped into the jungle, and I pray, I actually pray, for her to hold on until help arrives. Around my parents, I try to act normal. How to tell them what I'm feeling without telling everything? All I say is that I knew a lot of people in Peoples Temple, which is the truth, but not all of it.

Finally, I remember that Diane gave me her mother's phone number in Oakland, to use only in an absolute emergency. My hands shake as I dial the number.

"Hello, my name's Martina. I'm a friend of Diane's from Ukiah."

I get no further before she wails into the phone. "All my babies are gone, they're all gone." She's lost not only Diane, but also both of Diane's children and Diane's siblings.

All I can do is murmur "I'm so sorry" over and over as we sob together on the phone.

LIMBO

After our September 14th wedding, Tanya and I wait for the second opinion from Stanford. The next day, we drive up to Calistoga for our honeymoon, all the while keeping my cell phone on, even when I'm soaking in the tubs, waiting for the call that doesn't come. We return home to Cooper, who's living in the cottage in our backyard, and continue the wait.

On a Friday night two weeks after the wedding, as we head into another weekend, I'm discouraged that the doctor from Stanford still hasn't called. Even though I know that things with the medical establishment almost never happen when I think they should, not knowing his suggestions is depressing.

The phone rings. Tanya answers. "Yes, yes, she's here."

It's the surgeon calling from Stanford. We talk for half an hour. My notes of the conversation cover seven pages. Bottom line: Aggressive monitoring. No more surgery. No chemo.

When I hang up, I melt into Tanya's arms, so full of gratitude I can barely contain it. Cooper is grinning, but still worried. "How do we know it's gone? Are they sure?"

And the answer is: We don't know. Nothing is certain. But we hope so.

—

Which all sounds fine and good. Be in the moment. But what happens when you wake up the next morning from a long, vivid dream in which your Stanford surgeon is yelling at your Oakland surgeon while you're sitting there watching? When you wake up, you realize that you need to fire your Oakland surgeon. It's long overdue. You can no longer work with him. And all the fury you've sat on, all the tongue-biting you've done, is over. You're furious at him beyond words and write him a letter to tell him he's fired. You tell him how it felt when he routinely failed to respond to your phone calls or emails. You tell him how stressful it was when he failed to provide basic information to the Blue Cross billing department and Blue Cross wrote you that you would be responsible for thousands of dollars for your surgeries. You tell him how hard it is to trust him when he strongly advocates chemotherapy one week and then completely changes his mind one week later when you tell him the recommendation from Stanford is against chemotherapy. And finally, you berate his total nonchalance, in fact, his complete silence, about the loss of all the tissue from the surgery, tissue with no biopsy results because he failed to get it to the lab.

You send the letter by fax, marked "Personal," and immediately know that things could have been more artfully phrased. There could have been those so-called "I" messages, and fewer you, you, you messages. But you don't really care because you have been nice, nice, nice for *way* too long.

"There's no future, only now," our therapist says to Tanya and me. "That's how I cope. It works sometimes."

I think about it a moment. Until now I haven't detected any Buddhist leanings. This is new. "If there's just now," I say, "it's much harder to worry."

And every time I begin to worry, I take a breath and notice what's around me, and I'm calm, at least for the moment.

Still, the fact is, being in post-treatment mode is not easy. I'm past the stage of people bringing food; of supportive emails; of loving get-well cards. Everyone else is as tired of my health as I am. At this point, it's actually boring. Talking about it is boring. Thinking about it is boring. Going to endless appointments is boring. Even now, most weeks are filled with medical appointments.

The simple question of when to go back to work is fraught. My brain feels like oatmeal with raisins. The idea of sitting between two people who are getting a divorce and wrapping my radiated brain around their emotions, their finances, their kids, their budgets, and being competent—it's all overwhelming!

So I practice living in limbo. Not knowing what's next. Living day-by-day, moment-by-moment, looking for joy wherever I can find it. I suddenly remember a book about cancer that I was interviewed for in 1994: *Dancing in Limbo: Making Sense of Life after Cancer.* The author got my name as a cancer survivor and talked to me about my experience after treatment. The truth is, my recovery the first time wasn't extremely difficult, perhaps because I was much younger, had a new baby, and started a new career. I just moved ahead in life. But the book contains stories of people who had a rougher time and I feel compelled to look at it. I find the book at the very back of the bookcase, and I open it at random, like a true believer seeking solace from the *Bible.*

The words comfort me. I'm right on track. I've been through this before. Millions of us go through what I'm going through. I'm not alone. At my wedding, I vowed to dance as much as possible. I wasn't thinking of this particular dance at the time. I was thinking West Coast swing, rumba, and salsa. But this limbo dance is really the only dance there is.

STUCK IN THE LAND OF EST

I t's the fall of 1978. I climb the stairs of a tiny office building next to St. Mary's Square in San Francisco's Financial District and open the door to the only office on the second floor. Everything is sleek, expensive, subdued. Floor-to-ceiling windows look out over the city. Down the hill is the fifty-two-story Bank of America building where I worked nearly ten years ago. Cable car tracks run up the hill outside.

A woman greets me and introduces herself as Julie. She's stylishly dressed, made up, wearing high heels. "Jerry will be with you in a moment," she says. "Have a seat."

I sit in the waiting room, intimidated, wondering what in the world I'm doing in this place. I know I don't belong here.

I'm a hippie from Mendocino County. I live in San Francisco during the week, attending law school. David lives and works in Mendocino County full-time and we see each other on weekends. All I have to my name is our small cabin on fifty acres outside Ukiah, an old, white 1967 Ford Mustang, three pairs of drawstring pants, two turtlenecks, a couple of T-shirts, and sandals. And now my brand-new professional outfit—an incredibly uncomfortable turtleneck sweater with a scratchy wool blazer, slacks, and real shoes that I bought at Macy's in Santa Rosa just to wear to this meeting today.

I'm in my second year of law school and in desperate need of a paid internship. My study buddy Tom referred me to Jerry. "He's a gay lawyer I know," Tom said. "He's an EST fanatic, which you'll have to overlook. He's also a snob, but at least the job pays." EST stands for Erhard Seminars Training, a so-called personal growth experience that emphasizes "personal responsibility" and "creating your own reality." I'm desperate for a clerkship that pays because David earns too much for me to qualify for work-study, but not enough to pay my expenses. I *have* to work. So I'll overlook the EST connection. EST is an organization for which I have no respect. Its members seem phony, self-centered, and too ready to blame the poor for their problems.

Soon after Diane left Ukiah, it became clear to me that being a preschool teacher was not a great long-term career choice. Even though I loved the work, I earned only $350 per month, with almost no prospect of earning more unless I became an administrator, which didn't appeal to me. I loved the children, not paperwork and writing grants for funding.

That left me wondering what career to pursue. I had my BS from Southern Oregon and my teaching credential, but I needed more. I had already nixed being a public school teacher. Should I become a nurse? No, I'd have to take orders from doctors. Therapist? No, there were hundreds of female therapists in Mendocino County. Lawyer? Bingo. In 1976, there were only two women lawyers in the entire county!

I applied to three law schools in San Francisco. When I was accepted, I visited all three before making a choice. Hastings prided itself on having retired law professors on their faculty. When I looked in the catalogue, I saw a lot of older white men and almost no women. The class I sat in on was boring. Golden Gate sounded good on paper, but when I arrived, every single room was filled with smoke. I was a hippie from the country; I didn't want to choke on dirty air. When I arrived at New College, one of my idols, Susan Jordan, was teaching Criminal Law. Susan had developed a self-defense case for a woman accused of killing her rapist sometime after the rape had occurred. Experts testified about the impact of rape and the jury acquitted Inez Garcia, believing she was in fear when she committed the act. The students at New College were diverse, engaged, young, and rowdy. It was an easy choice, even though it was more expensive than Hastings.

Going to law school was a huge leap for me, so David and I decided that he would keep his job in Ukiah until I was sure law school was a match; I didn't want to be responsible for yet another move if studying law didn't work out. We'd moved enough in our eight years together—nine times, to be precise. We would have to see each other on weekends.

I joined a San Francisco commune in a huge Victorian just above Market and Castro, sharing space with six other people, including Bill Segen, the cable car driver from our commune in 1969.

The only available "room" when I moved in was in the eaves of the attic, with just enough space for a double futon, a little desk, and a dresser. A tiny window looked out over the rooftops at a sliver of lights sparkling in the distance. I was so happy to be in law school with a big goal that the transition wasn't problematic. And there's something to be said about weekend romance.

To my surprise, Jerry Berg hired me on Tom's recommendation after a brief phone interview. Today, I'm meeting him for the first time and reporting on my first assignment: my research on the legality of laetrile as a treatment for cancer. I enjoyed researching alternative health remedies since I'm a fan of herbs and non-Western medicine.

I worked hours on my memo, typed it up perfectly, and now I'm waiting to meet with Jerry. He strides in, one of the beautiful people—buffed, manicured, impeccably dressed, with a big insincere smile over perfectly straight white teeth. He barely shakes my hand before leading me into his meticulous office, where he reads my memo.

"How long did this take you?" he asks.

"About twenty hours," I answer honestly.

"How long *should* it have taken?"

"I don't know. Maybe five or six hours." My heart is pounding.

"I'll bill the client for six hours," he says. "Don't you think I should pay you for six hours, too?"

He looks deeply into my eyes and smiles what I will soon learn is the sincere EST gaze, and I know what to say if I want to keep the job. I nod meekly.

Within a month, I realize that I'm not going to make enough money working for Jerry to support myself. Not the way he counts hours. But I need the job to get my internship hours, so I decide to do what all my downwardly mobile, college-educated San Francisco housemates do: drive a bus. None of us would think about taking corporate jobs.

I get up at 4 a.m. every weekday morning, drive my car to the bus lot south of Market Street, pick up my bus, drive thirty minutes south to Foster City, pick up commuters, drive them into the Financial District, drop off my bus in the bus yard, and get to school or work by 8:30 in the morning.

I feel competent and powerful, maneuvering my bus in downtown San Francisco during rush hour. But I also feel stressed. Every morning I stare in my rearview mirror at a sea of faces nodding off or reading the *Chronicle* or a paperback or drinking coffee. All trusting me to get them safely to work.

Jerry telephones. "Can you come to a staff meeting at 9:00 on Tuesday morning?" This is a big deal. Until now, he has given me projects, but I don't work in the office or have a desk there, and I've never been asked to attend an office conference.

The day of the meeting I do my typical morning commute. The

temperature is approaching ninety when I arrive at the bus yard at the end of my shift. As I pump the bus with diesel fuel, it slushes onto my arm, but I don't have a moment to clean up if I'm going to arrive at work on time.

I trudge up the California Street hill, still wearing my bus driver uniform—a blue Oxford shirt, royal blue work pants, and Famolare sandals. Barely on time, hot and sweaty, smelling of diesel fuel, I dread being surrounded by Those-Who-Don't-Sweat.

Julie the receptionist looks perfect, as usual—makeup in place, fingernails painted, hair stylish but carefree. David the assistant looks preppy, alert, and efficient—notebook in hand, sharpened pencil behind his ear, legs crossed. Both are seated around Jerry's hardwood desk, an empty, glossy oval.

Jerry the boss makes his grand entrance, white teeth flashing, perfectly groomed in an elegant suit. Jerry, Julie, and David are all graduates of EST. Jerry is very busy creating success. Julie and David are very busy helping him.

Jerry takes his seat, smiles around the table, and says, "Martina, we are so happy you could come today. I can't pay you for this time, but I appreciate your coming, because I have an announcement to make." I marvel at how he can be so cheap. It would have cost $10 for my time today.

Jerry buzzes the intercom. "I just hired an associate, Tanya Starnes, and here she is." He grins, looking deeply at each of us, one by one. EST people are big on eye contact.

Through the door walks Tanya. Her long, blond hair falls loosely down her back below her waist. She's wearing a burgundy cashmere sweater dress, which clings to her body as if she were a model. Her feet are adorned in matching Fuck Me Pumps. She's definitely not sweating. She sits gracefully in the remaining chair, smiles at every-one, and speaks what seems to be perfect EST: "I am so happy to be here. This is a wonderful opportunity." Blah. Blah. Blah. All with a tinge of a Southern accent. I recognize that accent, subtle as it is at the moment. Both of my parents are from the South, and all of my cousins and extended family are still there. Not to mention that I spent many years in Virginia as a child. The South is steeped in my bones.

Jerry says, "Now, this is how things will work. Martina will work with Tanya, and David and Julie will work with me. Tanya will also have her own secretary, who will start soon."

I smile my best fake EST smile and welcome Tanya to the staff, all the while thinking: Please don't tell me I have to work with this woman. I can't do this.

LET'S HAVE A NORMAL LIFE

It's early October 2008 and Obama is running for president. I'm in my post-treatment limbo stage and desperate to be back in my normal life. Months of surgery and radiation have taken a toll. I yearn for something besides medical appointments in my calendar.

"Tanya's going to Florida or Ohio to do some Obama work," I tell Marjorie, our good friend, on our way back from Sunday breakfast at the Brown Sugar Kitchen. We've just gorged on grits, barbequed shrimp, and beignets. I've assumed that after Tanya and I had talked about the Obama campaign's need for help that Tanya would volunteer.

"I don't know what you're talking about," Tanya says.

I feel my chest constrict. For several months, I've been running a scenario in which Tanya would be our family contribution since I'm not strong enough to do a lot of precinct-walking myself. After ten months fighting cancer, I don't have the energy to do much of anything, but I still want to feel like I'm participating.

After Marjorie leaves, Tanya and I have a huge fight, the first since our wedding in September.

"But you've *got* to go," I say. "If I had the strength and energy and good health, I'd go myself. But you know I can't handle it." I'm in tears.

"I'm not going," she says. "The whole thing gives me a stomachache."

I can't believe that Tanya doesn't want to work on the campaign. I know she supports Obama. Why doesn't she want to do something? "I'm sorry about your stomachache. Mine is in knots, too," I say. Then, I get a little crazy. "But you can either watch the right wing take power, or fight them, but you can't sit on the sidelines with a stomachache." I'm shrieking now, but she won't budge.

A few days later, I learn that the campaign needs lawyers to watch the polls to ensure that everyone gets to vote. I figure that this is something I *can* do. I can pour out energy for one single day, even if I'll pay the price for a few days afterward.

Still prickly from our fight, I tell Tanya, "I'm going to Florida to be a poll watcher for the Obama campaign." It doesn't occur to me to see if she wants to go.

"I'll go with you," she says.

I can't figure out what's changed. Then I learn that it's not that Tanya didn't want to work on the campaign; it's that she's been stuck to me like an appendage for ten months, nursing me, driving me to appointments, cooking healthy food. She's not about to leave me for a week. I'm embarrassed. I'm supposed to be the professional communicator, the person who listens carefully to what everyone has to say when a conflict arises. I missed everything she was worried about. She's perfectly happy to be a poll watcher, too.

After several email conversations with the Obama campaign, it's decided that we'll go to Ohio, where we're needed more than in Florida.

We arrive in Columbus on November 1. The next morning, the Internet sends us to Poland, Ohio, via two-lane country roads instead of the freeway, and we meander through winding, hilly farm country dotted with occasional small towns. The yellows, reds, and oranges of fall remind me of the forests of my childhood in Virginia and New England. Red barns. Shimmering lakes. I notice, with knots in my stomach, more signs for McCain than for Obama.

Eventually, we reach Poland, Ohio, just south of Youngstown, home to miles and miles of strip malls, fast-food restaurants, and Kmarts. Concrete with no landscaping. We check into a Holiday Inn Express and settle in to read the inch-thick batch of materials from the campaign. By early evening, we need sustenance and find an Italian restaurant in the hotel literature. After Tanya tastes and rejects, with considerable embarrassment, the second of two possible white wines, the bartender comes over to talk. He's in his late twenties, blond, well-groomed, and friendly. He helps Tanya pick a beer and then tells us about the local scene when he learns we're from the Bay Area.

"I moved here from Florida to go to Youngstown State University. It's different here." He tells us that he's a Republican, but fed up with what's happening, so he's going to vote for Obama. He's bartending and in school getting a master's degree. His wife, a first-year teacher, earns $18,000 per year, and they can't afford to have a child. If she takes time off, they can't survive.

"Have you been to Youngstown yet?" he asks.

"No. We asked at the hotel where the downtown was for Poland, and the clerk said there *was* no downtown. So, we asked about the downtown for Youngstown, and she said there was no downtown there, either."

"Tomorrow," he says, "you should drive up to Youngstown. Just drive north on Market Street. Don't get on the freeway. Drive Market Street. You'll see. It's a ghost town." He tells us that there used to be 200,000 people living in Youngstown. Now there are 45,000. The population is shrinking seven percent per year. There are no jobs. The GM plant is the only big one still open. The only thing in Youngstown that's thriving is YSU.

The next morning, we drive to Youngstown, and despite the heads-up from the bartender, we're totally unprepared for what we see. The term Rust Belt takes on new meaning. Blocks and blocks of boarded-up homes; eighty percent of businesses closed; huge factories empty; barges rusting on the river. Nothing vibrant and alive for miles except YSU and two federal buildings. It seems like this is the heart of the campaign, all that Obama has been talking about. The hopelessness is pervasive.

We drive back to Poland to the Obama headquarters to train for poll watching. The license plates on the cars in the parking lot are from Pennsylvania, Rhode Island, Kentucky, California, Virginia, West Virginia, New York. I tear up, thinking of all these people coming such distances to do this work. This is the first time I've been a part of something bigger than my cancer and myself for a long time.

As we check in, the Obama worker says, "I need to know that you will be working all day tomorrow."

I have a moment of panic about whether I can actually *do* what I've committed to do. Even though it's only one very long day, I'm worried about my energy. I'm still very depleted. Not to mention that I can barely text, and all communication from today forward will be by text.

I nod yes, anyway.

We find a spot at the back of the room, open our folders, and see with relief that both Tanya and I are assigned to the same place, Milton Lake fire station.

The trainers announce that there are 4,500 volunteer lawyers in Ohio and 5,800 in Florida, all prepared to deal with problems as they arise and ensure that everyone gets to vote. The organization is unbelievable. "When this training is over, we want you to go find your assigned polling place while it's daylight, so you're not wandering around at 5 a.m., trying to find your spot."

Back through the Ohio countryside, thirty minutes from Youngstown, we arrive at our assignment in Milton Lake. It's idyllic. Rolling hills, a serene lake, farms, tidy trailer parks. We're a bit disappointed not to be in an urban area, but we figure that the campaign knows what it's doing.

On Election Day, our alarm beeps at 4:45 a.m. At precisely 5:00, Tanya's cell phone rings with a robocall from John Kerry, telling us to get up and get going. Thirty minutes later, we hit the lobby and find two other lawyers doing the same thing we're doing—dragging our tired bodies out into the dark, cold morning to be at the polls at 5:45 a.m. The sweet smell of four dozen Dunkin' Donuts wafts from the back seat of the car. We figured we might as well take treats. The trunk is loaded with warm coats and food to last all day.

When we arrive at the Milton Lake fire station, poll workers are already pulling into the lot. By 6:15, there's a line of fifteen or twenty voters. They all know each other. By 6:34, when the three precinct desks inside open up four minutes late, there are fifty people in line outside, where it's still very dark and freezing cold.

We have no way to discern whether we're helping McCain supporters or Obama supporters. These Ohio folks don't display their allegiances. We simply help every person who comes to the firehouse find the right line, have the correct ID, and get organized to vote.

It's dark as we wait for the votes from our three precincts to be tallied. Obama wins all three by a substantial margin! By 10:00 p.m., we've successfully texted on Tanya's Blackberry, a major feat for us, all the required information to the Obama headquarters. Back at our hotel, the TV is on, and when Ohio gets called for Obama, we're ecstatic.

All I want to do is sleep, I am utterly spent, but I make myself stay up with Tanya for Obama's speech. Tears stream down our faces the entire time.

—

The next day, Tanya and I drive back to Columbus and stop at a gas station near the airport to fill our rental car. In front of us is a rickety old Chevrolet, rusted and funky. A skinny black man in a black baseball cap is pumping gas with his back to us.

"It's a great morning, isn't it?" Tanya says to him.

The man turns around and I can see OBAMA written across the front of his baseball cap.

"We came from California to work for Obama," I hear Tanya tell him.

They fall into each other's arms, hugging and laughing, and as Tanya turns to deal with our gas pump, I see that she's crying.

"Thanks for helping us," the man calls as we drive away.

Two days after the election, we're back in Berkeley. Everyone is beaming about Obama, but I'm lost in a fog of grief that Proposition 8, California's anti-gay marriage proposition, might pass. I'm home alone while Tanya gets our dog, Mollie, from her mother.

Despite the evidence I see on the TV, I cling to the possibility that the early votes and absentee ballots, when counted, will change the bad outcome. The venom and lies of the anti-gay marriage campaign shocked me: phone calls to African Americans to tell them that Obama wanted them to vote against gay marriage; legal "scholars" telling voters that the state would require their church to perform gay weddings or lose its tax-exempt status; ads telling parents that their children would be taught gay marriage in school.

Late in the morning, I receive an email from the National Center for Lesbian Rights that says it's over. Prop 8 has passed and marriage is limited to one man and one woman.

I read the email and weep.

I wander through the house, looking for Kleenex and solace. I only find the Kleenex. Slowly, I become furious. Why didn't I see this coming? Why did we spend our money on a wedding? Even though our marriage will likely remain legal, this vote against same-sex marriage is a huge loss. I feel horrible that we didn't donate the money from our September wedding to the fight against Proposition 8. We knew Prop 8 was looming when we got married.

All the progressive organizations I belong to are sending emails celebrating Obama's victory, without even mentioning this crushing loss, and how it might feel to those of us most immediately affected by it.

But a few hours later, I get emails from my friends Maude and Dana, expressing their grief about Prop 8. Our neighbors, all straight couples, come over to our house to express their condolences.

Tanya and I wander down to O Chame, our favorite restaurant, for some healthy nourishment, since our refrigerator is bare from our trip to Ohio. Our friend Ivette is picking up food to go and drops by our table.

"How are you two?" she asks.

I smile and automatically say, "Fine." Then, I catch myself and tell the truth. "Actually, I'm not fine. I'm so unhappy about Prop 8."

"I know," she says. "Every lesbian I've run into is the same way. Me too. It's been really hard being sad with all the Obama euphoria."

The final tally: 6,313,674 Californians voted to protect the rights of animals to have cages large enough to move around in. But only 4,932,086 voted to protect the rights of the LGBTQ community.

I stay angry for several days more before I give it up and move on. Anger's not good for the soul—or the immune system.

YOU'RE STRAIGHT?

It's the fall of 1979 when I begin assisting Tanya at work, coming into the office only when I need to meet with her to discuss assignments. The work is practical. "Look at the file and write a status letter to the client." "Research the statute of limitations for fraud."

I do the work, return the file to her, and she reviews it. My work always comes back to me marked up. If I have a long, elegant sentence, she cuts it up into three curt sentences. "Martina, you have to write these letters like you're talking to *idiots,* even when you're writing for the court," she says. "Simple sentences. Subject. Verb. Object. New sentence. Don't be insulted. Your work is fine. I just want it my way." She talks like she writes. No nonsense, no fluff.

We work like this for several months, knowing nothing about each other.

One Friday afternoon, I hand her an assignment. "I have to leave quickly," I say. "I'm driving up to Ukiah to see my husband for the weekend."

"You're *married?*" she yelps.

"Yes, I thought you knew that." I'm laughing at the look on her face.

"To a man?" She's bewildered.

"Yes, to David."

"I thought you were a lesbian."

"I take that as a compliment," I say, "but I'm not."

Tanya tells me that her roommate is Betsy Belote and now it's my turn to be shocked.

"I know Betsy," I say. "I took a women's assertiveness training class from her in 1973." I can't help wondering what Betsy, an obvious lesbian, is doing living with this straight girl for a roommate. It makes no sense.

Several months later, Tanya invites me to dinner. After work, I ride with her in her blue VW bug to her house on Arguello near Golden Gate Park. Thick burgundy carpet covers the stairs to the second-floor flat. Velvet-flocked wallpaper shimmers on the walls. It feels like a Victorian whorehouse. I've never been in any place like it.

Betsy meets us at the top of the stairs in blue jeans and a work shirt and gives me a tour. "This is Tanya's bedroom," she says.

I peek into a small room with a single bed and a white lace bedspread reminiscent of my bedroom in the sixth grade. Nothing is out of place.

"This is my bedroom," she says. Betsy's bedroom is down the hall, with a very small double bed.

There's a woodstove in the kitchen, an old-fashioned fireplace in the living room, and prim and proper velvet-upholstered Victorian furniture.

Betsy and Tanya are completely restoring the flat themselves. They work on it weekday mornings before work; Betsy then drives Tanya to the office by 8:00 and returns home to her therapy practice. Each evening and every weekend, they continue with their projects. I'm amazed by their energy.

"I don't know why Betsy pretends that I have my own bedroom," Tanya says the next week at work. "We never sleep in it. We sleep in her room."

It's my turn to yelp. "You mean you're a couple?"

"Didn't you know that?"

"I didn't know you were a lesbian."

"I fool a lot of people," she grins.

Eventually, Tanya and I reveal to each other that we both loathe EST and sneak off for espressos at the coffee house down the street just to get away from the office. It's stressful smiling and creating success all the time.

"You want to know what Jerry gave me for a Christmas bonus?" she asks. "A beautiful card with a coupon in it. He wanted to pay one-half of the tuition for an introductory EST program."

"What did you do?"

"I asked him in my best EST-talk whether I could have the money instead. He said, 'No, that's not what I had in mind. I thought you would benefit from the program. I'm giving you half the tuition. You pay the other half, so you're enrolled in the process.'" Being "enrolled" is EST-talk for being committed, which is very important to Jerry.

"So, what are you going to do?" I ask.

"I declined the gift. You should have seen the expression on his face."

Betsy decides to treat Tanya, David, and me to dinner at a fancy restaurant in Napa Valley for Tanya's twenty-seventh birthday in August of 1980. I'm delighted that Tanya wants to spend her birthday with us. By now, she and I have become good friends, and our partners seem to like each other.

Betsy is a Ph.D. psychologist, a contractor, and a writer. David is still the director of the Mendocino County Youth Project. A practicing Buddhist, he's begun studying with an old Chinese master who's the head of the City of 10,000 Buddhas, a Buddhist temple that bought the California state hospital in Talmage outside Ukiah. Monks and nuns live on the grounds, translate old Chinese Buddhist texts into English, and study with their master.

Betsy and David chatter about intellectual and spiritual matters. They go on and on, while Tanya and I are very quiet. After a while, I look across the table and see that she's profoundly bored.

We pass a look to each other, and I interject, "Hey, you two, we want to tell you about how things are at work." I know, by now, that Tanya will be hilarious.

"Here's how we do file review." Tanya laughs. "We sit around Jerry's polished desk and wait quietly for Jerry. He always manages to make a grand entrance after all of us are seated and waiting. When he arrives, he sits and folds his perfectly manicured hands like this." Tanya clasps her hands, sits ramrod straight, and puts on her best EST smile. "Jerry looks around the table and says, 'Who would like to share first?' Then he looks sincerely at each of us, one at a time, until someone starts. Everybody has to share something and it has to be *meaningful*. When each person is done, he says, 'Thank you for sharing.' Big smile. David the assistant has a card for each of our cases. He sits forward over crossed legs, with his two perfectly sharpened no. 2 pencils, ready to make notes on each case.

"As far as I can tell," Tanya continues, "Jerry is in charge of nothing but file review. He has never done work on a single case. Either David is doing the work, or Julie is making a phone call, or Martina is doing research, or I'm figuring out what to do. And God help us if two weeks go by and one of us hasn't done what we were supposed to according to file review notes."

The longer Tanya talks, the more her Southern accent turns on. Storytelling brings it on strong.

"How about the Hunger Project?" I say, goading her on.

"They actually get people to pay money to go to seminars where they sit and have the *intention* to end world hunger," Tanya says.

"They don't do anything about it. They just have the intention. It's worse than the Baptist preachers I grew up with."

Finally, we do our routine about the money: Jerry pays me $5.00 per hour and bills my time to his clients at $35 per hour; he pays Tanya $25 per hour and bills her time at $125 per hour.

By the end of the evening, we've exhausted ourselves from good food, wine, and laughter.

A month later, I start my last year of law school and decide to intern in a criminal law office to get more experience. I'm making good money as a bus driver now and can afford to volunteer with lawyers I want to learn from. But I worry about telling Tanya that I'm leaving. I call my study buddy Tom, who referred me to Jerry, to talk it over.

"I feel loyal to Tanya," I say. "She's spent hours training me. I'm good at it now, and she'll have to start all over with someone else."

"You have to take care of yourself," Tom says. "They paid you five dollars an hour *because* you were an intern. Interns leave, by definition. Stop feeling guilty."

Easier said than done. I take the easy way out, still feeling like a traitor: I quit on a day that Tanya's not there and leave her a note. She calls me on my home phone the next night.

"Martina, I can't *believe* you're leaving me! What are you *thinking*? Now I'm here all alone." The words are harsh, but she's laughing. "Don't worry. I totally understand. It's okay."

Within a month, I hear that Tanya has quit, too, and opened her own office on Hayes Street in San Francisco.

STALKING THE RAT

Tanya and I are cocooned in our bed on the second floor of the house at 5 a.m. in November, just after Obama's election; the house is pitch black and freezing cold because the furnace hasn't gone on yet. It's on a timer to go on at 6:30 a.m.

PLOP! There's a noise coming from the kitchen.

Tanya sneaks downstairs in her T-shirt, turns on the light, and yells, "It's a rat!" I run down and see an apple from the counter, now on the floor with little bites chunked out of one side. I can see the little teeth marks!

"Where is it?" I ask.

"Under the stove," she says.

I go back upstairs and bring her a robe and slippers.

We have to leave early for an appointment at Stanford to get a PET scan today, so I go back upstairs to get ready. Tanya wants to shoo the rat out and stands guard in the kitchen.

When I come downstairs again after my shower, Tanya has laid a trail of treats that stretches from the stove to the wide-open back door. Icy wind whips through the house as she stands there with a broom, waiting to encourage the rat out the door. "It waddles like Ratatouille," she says. Apparently, it ventured forth once, before realizing she was there.

I bundle up and make breakfast for us while she stands there for another hour. The rat peeks out several times and runs back under the stove until we finally have to leave for Palo Alto.

—

The PET scan involves injecting radioactive material into my arm. It attaches to both cancer and to inflammation. The results: an area in my neck lights up. Because it's in the area where they already operated for cancer, it could be a recurrence or just inflammation. The plan: an MRI in a few weeks to distinguish between inflammation and cancer. The impact: more waiting before we'll know what's going on.

I send an email to my cancer list, a list of all the friends and family who want to keep up with what is going on with my illness. I periodically send updates to reduce the number of phone calls and explanations I have to make. It's just too hard talking to people on an individual basis. In this email, I describe the results of the PET scan and tell them that my intuition is that everything will be okay since I've been feeling so good. Then, to add a little humor, I write a riff about the rat and Tanya lining up the treats to lure it out the door.

Our friend Liz writes back: "I'm sorry for the ongoing delay in leaving this phase behind. I will meditate on the rat finding a new home, and on the picture of the treats Tanya laid out for him/her. I didn't know Texans were so humane and friendly; I'd have thought she'd just shoot it, and the linoleum, too."

Our friend Debby writes back: "Stalking the cancer, stalking the rat; seems like you guys should be getting a break right about now."

I agree. I'm weary. We've had enough bad news.

The truth is, when I wrote the email to my friends, I *did* feel optimistic. But a day later, bubbles of anxiety rise from my gut like hot air balloons. Fear radiates in waves, followed by nausea. What if I'm not going to make it this time?

"I don't want to kill the rat," I say. "Let's use one of those humane traps that won't kill it."

Cooper, the environmentalist, agrees.

Tanya buys a humane trap at the hardware store, puts peanuts inside, and leaves it along the wall in the living room at the spot where we think the rat comes in. The next morning, it has walked right around the trap. Instead of going for the goodies, it went to the kitchen door and began to gnaw a hole through it to get to Mollie's dog food on the other side! Little wood chips lie scattered on the floor.

"This isn't working," Tanya says. "I think the person who's getting rid of the rat should pick the method. I'm getting a rat zapper to shock and kill it."

The zapper's directions say that you have to be patient, that it might take up to ten days before the rat goes inside, takes the bait, and gets zapped.

Meanwhile, the little sucker is having a party every night.

I've barely worked since I was diagnosed in January, and now, eleven months later, after two surgeries and seven weeks of radiation, I have only a few clients left. Several attorneys begged me to help them finish a divorce mediation before the end of the year. I was reluctant. I don't like to mediate with lawyers in the room; I just want to work with the couple. Not to mention that I don't even know how well my brain works at this point. It feels mushy, unclear, spaced. But I agreed, and today's the day of the meeting.

Since I've already given up my office on Fourth Street, the five of us—the couple, the two lawyers, and I—are meeting in my home office at my antique round, wooden table. For over an hour, we talk about assets and finances.

Finally, we need a break, and as I open the office door, the wife calmly says, "Martina, do you have a pet rat?"

Here I am, trying to be professional in a less-than-professional setting, and the frigging rat takes a stroll across the hallway into the other office where my assistant Kim usually works! Fortunately, Kim's not here now. The wife's lawyer, dressed elegantly, perfectly coiffed, and made up, rolls her eyes and lifts her feet.

I jump up and slam the door to Kim's office, stuffing a towel in the gap underneath so the rat can't come back out in our direction.

"Well, I didn't have a rat until a few days ago," I say, totally mortified as I describe how we bought a gas insert for our fireplace and the installation left a small opening to the outside that provided the access for the rat to get in the house.

"Now are you motivated to let me get the rat any way I can?" Tanya asks after she hears what happened during the mediation.

"Okay," I say, leaving all my lofty principles behind.

Tanya buys ten old-fashioned rat traps and distributes them in the basement and living room.

A few days later, she's resting at the kitchen table. Her hair is sticking straight up from wearing a bicycle helmet in the basement. Why a bicycle helmet in the basement? So she won't bang her head on the joists while she's patching rat holes. This is *so* Tanya, I find myself laughing.

"Can I ask you a question?" I say. "I don't want you to freak out."

She looks up at me and nods.

"Have you thought about me dying this time?" I start to cry. "I don't want you to be alone."

"Don't worry," she says, "I'll have the rats." Her gentle blue eyes seek mine. "I thought about it at the beginning, but right now I'm thinking the PET scan is showing inflammation," she says. "And if I weren't covered in rat turds and dirt, I'd hug you."

That night, Cooper heads out to the cottage in our backyard, which we turned into a small studio for him to live in after graduation from college while he gets on his feet. I'm ready to turn on the alarm system and lock the house for the night when I hear a quiet tapping at the back door. I look out into the darkness, and there he is, smiling at me. I open the door and he gives me a huge hug without saying a word.

We're all waiting and worrying about what the MRI will reveal.

On the Monday before Thanksgiving, the MRI shows more cancer. And despite knowing fully well that this was a possibility, I still feel bludgeoned.

"How soon can you operate?" I ask.

"Maybe Wednesday," the doctor says.

"You get a medal if you can do it Wednesday," Tanya says, "and I can get out of cooking for Thanksgiving."

On Thanksgiving Day, rather than sitting around a table piled with food, I'm in a stupor from the surgery I'd indeed opted to have the day before. The surgeon cut out more tumors, lymph nodes, and muscle from my neck. Tanya sits in a chair across the room in her own stupor from sleeping on the world's most uncomfortable cot.

Four doctors stride into the room. They probe, look in my mouth, ask me to smile.

"You're doing fine."

"Can you answer a question?" I ask.

"Sure." The lead doctor is young, very good-looking, attentive, warm.

"Were you there for the surgery?"

"Yes."

"Can you tell me about it? I don't remember talking to my surgeon yesterday."

"We worked a long time," he says. "Seven hours. The main tumor was adhered to the carotid artery, and was scraped off."

"How big was it?"

He makes a fist and says, "About half that size."

For the first time, I feel terror. When the lead doctor comes back with the entourage at the end of the day, I say, "Can I talk to you a moment?" He's tied up but promises me he'll come back after they finish rounds.

"Are you giving me a death sentence?" I ask when he returns. He looks right at me. "No, I'm not," he says. "We got clean margins. We think we got it all. Now we just have to wait."

The next day, my friend and colleague Susan Flax peeks into my hospital room. A divorce mediator by profession, she volunteers with the Stanford chaplaincy program and mentioned she would stop by. I motion her in. I'm on lots of pain medication and consumed with anxiety about the size of the tumor. I tell Susan about it.

"I want to tell you a story," she says. "When I was a kid, my father was diagnosed with cancer on his shoulder. We lived in Ohio, and the local doctors said they couldn't handle it and sent him to Sloan Kettering." Thinking he would probably die, her father sold his business and made arrangements. At a family conference, he told her and her mother what he'd done to take care of things.

"He, my mother, and I went to Sloan Kettering," she continues. "I still remember the day before the surgery. My father looked at the surgeon with his big brown eyes and said, 'Doctor, do you have to remove my arm?' The doctor said, 'Probably so.' My dad looked at him and said, 'I guess that's okay.'"

After the surgery, she tells me, he looked like half the person he had been. His whole arm and shoulder were gone. She and her mother went to the hotel that night because he was sedated. Assuming that he would still be sedated, they didn't go back until late the next morning. When they walked in his room, he was sitting up, dressed in a work shirt, clean-shaven, and reading the newspaper.

"Where the hell have you been?" he said.

"He lived another thirty years," Susan says. "So you just never know."

When she slips out of the room, I feel soothed.

This time, I'm in a narcotic stupor for three weeks. The drugs make me sleep all the time. Even if I think of something I want to do, I don't have the energy to do it. Time passes. I imagine my death, my memorial service, life in my household without me. Tears flow randomly, without warning. At times, I'm at peace, gazing out the window at brilliant blue skies and leafless trees, feeling the golden afternoon light pouring over my bed where I doze.

My friend Leann comes to visit. Her son Jake is Cooper's close friend. Our families met years ago at Camp It Up family camp. She crawls right into bed with me, snuggling up and chattering away.

In early December, ten days after surgery, the surgeon tells me that the tumor they removed was bigger than they had anticipated. But the pathology report was better than expected, and most of the tissue they removed was negative for the tumor. The cancer was confined to one spot and stuck tightly to my carotid artery. They got clean margins there and everywhere else, which means they think they got all of the cancer. The future: monitoring every few months. I'm delighted with this news. Maybe surgery will work this time. I'm relieved to take off the medical pressure and prepare for the year-end holidays.

Meanwhile, the rat continues to taunt us. I think it would be fitting for us to have gotten rid of it by now. It's too much, rats gnawing our house and cancer gnawing my body. The rat has eluded sixteen traps of all varieties available on the market. It's smart, figures out how the traps work, and then avoids them. Tanya has sealed off holes and entry points into the house, so it's now confined to the attic and basement (we hope), with a freeway between them in the walls (which we haven't located yet).

The phrase "I smell a rat" takes on new meaning when Tanya goes into the basement one afternoon to do a rat check and comes back upstairs gasping.

"There must be a dead rat in the basement," she says. "And I'm not going to find it."

She gets our neighbor Paul, who brings his dog, Harley, who finds the rat quickly. Paul removes it for us.

Tanya is ecstatic, dancing around the house, chanting, "We got the rat. We got the rat." Maybe we're done with both the rat and the cancer.

But overnight, three chocolate decorations on the Christmas tree disappear. Where there's one rat, we quickly learn, there are more. In response to another email from me, emails pour in from friends with their personal rat solutions. One friend suggests putting talcum powder around spots where the rat could be coming in to see where he goes and what he does. Tanya clears the living room of rugs and miscellaneous stuff, leaving only the tree and sofas. She spreads talcum powder on the floor and behold, the next day, we see that the critter still comes in through the fireplace insert, but hangs high on the sides so it can walk above all the glue traps lining the floor around the fireplace. Little white footprints mark its path. This guy can climb, because he made his way across the room, up the slick sides of the black-lacquered grand piano, and into a bowl of potpourri. At some point he fell, and there in the talcum powder is his silhouette: seven inches long, not including the tail!

—

We have no intention of giving our house over to the rats, so we continue with our Christmas preparations. The living room is beautiful and sparkling. The tree is decorated with ornaments we brought with us from childhood and many more collected during our twenty-eight years together. Poinsettias splash red in white vases under the windows. The afternoon sun warms the room. Sitting on the couch, I have an unbidden thought: What if this is my last Christmas? Tears roll down my cheeks. When I tell Tanya why, she holds me in her arms and cries, too, as we cling to each other in front of the fire.

Just after the new year, Tanya wakes up full of energy and says, "I feel it, I'm going to catch a rat today." There's no reason she should think this. All we've gotten so far is the dead rat that Harley the dog found. But she's ever-optimistic.

After almost two months of setting traps, she's upped the ante with rat zappers placed outside along the perimeter of the house. She runs inside through the back door that night. "I think I got a rat in the rat zapper," she announces.

"What are we going to do?"

"I'm not going to take it out of the trap," she says.

We go out to look. "I can't do this either," I say. It's so embarrassing, being such sissies. We run to the front window to see if Paul is awake. His glowing TV gives us the good news, and Tanya sneaks across the street and knocks softly on his door so she won't wake his wife Bonnie. Paul quietly disposes of the dead rat, and we get two more over the next two nights, which Tanya proudly disposes of by herself.

We think we're finally done, but a few mornings later, Tanya says, "Come look."

She leads me into the attic, where another rat has gnawed a hole all the way through the plywood doors to feast on soap stored in the attic.

That night, she places a glue trap by the hole leading into the attic, and the next morning, she rushes into the bedroom completely horrified. "Oh, no, I didn't think this through. There's a rat in there, looking at me, stuck to the trap. It's squeaking. I can't do this." I *know* I can't do this. Paul is away, but Bonnie comes over with Paul's big gloves, sneaks a peek and says, "Not me."

What about Joe? Our next-door neighbor, he's an environmentalist. A poet. An arborist. He'll probably hate doing this worse than *we* do, but we're desperate. We call his house. "Oh, no problem," his wife, Anna, says. "Joe is good with stuff like this."

Joe comes over and goes straight up into the attic. When he comes out, he looks at me, rolls his eyes, and says, "Don't ask," as he leaves the house with a small bag. I know better than to ask what he's going to do with it.

We wonder. Could this finally be it?

Later in January, I have an appointment to review the MRI from the day before. While we're waiting, I read an obituary in the *San Francisco Chronicle* about a woman who was told she was dying in 1992 but didn't die for seventeen more years. These days, I appreciate obituaries like this.

My surgeon arrives. I show him some small bumps that look like little pimples on my neck, thinking they are nothing, but wanting to be certain.

He says, nonchalantly, "These are cancer."

"Can you operate on them? They're right on the top of the skin."

"No, because it won't help," he says. "It's a recurrence and they'll just keep appearing in other places. The only thing that can help slow things down now is chemotherapy. But we'll biopsy them to be certain."

"So, you're telling me I'm dying of this, right?"

"Yes."

"How long?"

"Maybe a year. You've probably got double digits of months left." The words pierce through me, but I feel oddly calm. I don't look at Tanya, who is madly taking notes.

The doctor leaves the room and we wait for the pathologists. We don't talk. We don't cry. We sit very, very still.

An hour passes before the pathologists arrive, three of them. They take biopsies of each little bump. Then my surgeon returns and, as a precaution, takes a bigger biopsy of one of them, as if to prove his point. Twenty minutes later, we're told that the preliminary report is negative for cancer, but there won't be a final report until later in the week.

We're both elated and utterly spent. How could he tell us I was dying when he didn't really know for sure?

On January 29, 2009, the phone rings in the morning.

"Hi, Martina. This is Shaun, one of your nurses from Stanford Clinic." I feel myself get tense, but I think that if the news were bad, the doctor would call me in person. "The final results of your pathology are positive. We put your case before the Tumor Board today and everyone agreed that you should see an oncologist and get chemotherapy. We've already talked to the oncologists, so you should get a call in a few days to schedule an appointment."

Tanya sits beside me on the couch and knows immediately what's happening. I hang up, blasted wide open. Time slows. Seconds seem like minutes. Cooper is in the kitchen, cooking. My assistant, Kim, is in our home office in the next room.

"Kim and Cooper!" I call out. "You need to come in here. I have to talk to you."

They walk into the room, faces ashen.

"The cancer has spread and I will probably die in the next year or two." I start to cry, and then we all start to cry. "I'm so sorry to put you all through this."

Later in the day, Cooper, Tanya, and I sit in our bedroom, catching some early afternoon sun. He tears up. "It's my fault you have cancer, Mom."

"Why do you say that?"

"Because when you first got diagnosed, I made a deal with God that if you were okay after the surgery, I'd stop smoking, and I didn't stop." He's crying now.

I walk across the room, smooth his hair, caress his forehead, and kiss the top of his head. "God doesn't work that way, Cooper. It's not your fault. I promise you that."

"Magical thinking," Tanya says.

"Everyone has magical thinking," I say. "Here's mine: I think I was supposed to get the message to close my business, but I didn't do it, so that's why it hasn't gone away."

Tanya says: "Here's mine. I think that if I had tried hard enough, I would have caught the rats sooner, and if I'd done that, the cancer would be gone."

I feel both intensely present in my life and as if I'm floating above it. I check my calendar and see that I have a late-afternoon appointment for a haircut, so I go and chat about the usual stuff with Angela, without even telling her what's going on.

When I come home, Cooper and Tanya are sitting in the living room together. He says, "I don't know how to think about this."

"It's really hard to both be thinking that I'm dying, and simultaneously holding hope that something will work or that there will be a miracle," I say. "I have trouble with it, too."

"That's just what I told him," Tanya says. "He asked what to tell his friends. 'Do I tell them my mother is dying?' And I said that we should tell the truth. The truth is, we don't know, but it doesn't look good. You're going to see oncologists to see what they have to say. The doctors aren't optimistic. But I told him about the group we went to after you had cancer when he was a baby, and how many of them had been told they were dying and didn't die."

After Cooper leaves for his cottage, Tanya and I are sitting in front of the fire on the couch when she suddenly bursts into tears and wails, gasping for air, grabbing me, clinging as if she's drowning. I hold her as tight as I can, tears noiselessly running down my cheeks. "I don't want you to leave me!" she screams, pounding the couch. "This isn't right."

By 8:30, she's sleeping softly next to me in our bed on our new flannel sheets and I'm reading my *New Yorker,* a blessed distraction that arrived in the mail today.

After sleeping like a baby, I wake up to the memory of the first time I told Tanya I loved her and start to cry. I shower, blow my hair dry, brush my teeth. I wonder if I should have my dental work done or just skip it. Then I figure I need more information to know whether or not to spend the money on my teeth.

We're lounging upstairs in our bedroom because in the winter, that's where the sun is, streaming in through the sliding glass doors. Cooper and Hayley, his girlfriend of several years, slam the front door.

"Mom!" he calls out.

"Cooper!" we call back.

"Can we come up?"

"Sure."

They climb the stairs and plop onto the couch at the foot of the bed.

"Any good news today?" he asks.

"Nothing, except we have appointments with oncologists on Wednesday and Friday next week."

"I think they made a mistake," he says.

A few days later, we go to Picante, our favorite spot to eat when we want something good, fast, and inexpensive. Fish tacos do the job. It feels like spring, but it's really the drought, which makes it almost sinful to enjoy the fresh, warm air.

"Will you do the rat check when we get home from lunch?" I ask Tanya.

"Sure."

The rat check means cruising through the attic to look for signs that a rat has been there, and then going into the basement to see if the peanuts she's left out have been taken. For almost three weeks, things have been untouched, and I'm ready to declare victory over the rats, if not the cancer.

Later, Tanya comes into my office while I'm writing and says, "One of the peanuts is gone."

"Are you certain?"

"Yes."

But as it turns out, Tanya is mistaken. The rats are finally gone, though it takes another few weeks for us to finally declare victory. Stalking the cancer continues, but at least we beat the rats.

FRACTURE LINES

By the fall of 1980, I'm in my last year of law school. It's the fourth year, because New College requires internships and practical experience, and it all can't get done in three years. I still live in my commune in San Francisco during the week and see David every weekend.

Our marriage, so strong until now, begins to feel fragile. Multiple fracture lines appear. David makes big changes: he leaves the Youth Project to become a priest again in the Episcopal Church in Ukiah. When I met him, he'd mostly left the church behind. During our time together, he's been a meditator and a Buddhist. I'm anguished by this move: being a priest's wife is *not* in my plan. I don't even consider myself a Christian. I'm a spiritual person, but I believe there are many ways to experience the divine, not just one. David is deeply engaged with his Christian friends and the church, from which I feel distant. In addition, our age difference, which hasn't mattered before, is now becoming an issue; I'm in my early thirties, ready to fly; he's in his early fifties, ready to settle down.

Since my experience with Diane, and particularly while I've been in law school, it's become clearer to me that I'm drawn to women. But I certainly don't want to leave my marriage.

We're both serious and thoughtful about our problems. We're very connected; we can talk about everything; we enjoy each other. A friend suggests that we read *Portrait of a Marriage* by Nigel

Nicholson, the son of Vita Sackville-West and Harold Nicholson. Nicholson's parents had a long and interesting marriage and a compelling intellectual relationship. Each of them took lovers throughout the marriage; one of Vita's was Virginia Woolf. David and I think our relationship will last forever, that our connection is enduring. Although I'm attracted to women, I can't imagine life without David.

We have friends in Ukiah who have children together and a strong marriage, but the wife also has relationships with women. We wonder if we can have a relationship like that and decide to try an open marriage. I have thoughts about one of the women at my law school who I think might be just right.

In early December, I'm having dinner with Tanya at Diamond Sutra, a restaurant off 24th Street in San Francisco, to prepare her for a mock trial at my law school. She has agreed to be a witness. We haven't worked together for many months, but we've stayed in touch. As we finish the trial prep, we move on to talking about our lives.

"I'm really upset," I say.

"Why?"

"It's a long story." I tell her that David and I have decided to try an open marriage and that I wanted to have a relationship with a woman from law school.

"She's the perfect person for me," I say. "We like each other a lot. She's in a committed relationship with her girlfriend; I'm committed to my marriage. But her girlfriend just decided she wasn't comfortable with it because they just moved here and aren't settled yet. My friend and I had coffee this afternoon and she said it isn't going to work. I feel like I'll never find the right person."

Tanya is laughing at me. "You had *coffee* to talk about an affair? What's *wrong* with you? If you're gonna have an affair, you go out to dinner with candles and wine. You don't *talk* about it. You're way too in your head, Martina."

I'm so in my head that I don't even notice that we're having dinner with candles and wine.

I tell her about David's new job. "It's distressing." By now, David and I have been together for eleven years. During this time, he's been a streetcar driver, an English teacher, a director of youth programs, and a devout Buddhist. Now, suddenly, he's embracing his Christianity. "I'm having a hard time with the church thing. And besides the church, it's even more problematic because he's gotten into a group that speaks in tongues."

Tanya rolls her eyes. Her hometown of Beaumont, Texas, was filled with tongue-speakers. She wants nothing to do with this kind of religion.

Bored with my own problems, I ask her how she's doing.

"I've split up with Betsy," she says, "and I'm hauling my stuff around in my VW." By now, she's been with Betsy three years. They've almost finished remodeling their Victorian. I'm surprised by this change.

"Where are you staying?"

"With friends. I'm going to Suzanne's place in Berkeley when she leaves for the holidays next week."

"Where are you going tonight?" I ask.

"I haven't figured that out," she says.

"Well, come home with me. There's extra space in our flat," I say, thinking of the living room couch. I have not one thought of romance on my mind.

She follows me to my flat.

And a few hours later, without any conscious intention on my part, I find myself in the same bed with her, entwined and thrilled.

HOPE

Three days before the 2008 election, my neighbor Joe, the arborist, poet, and rat catcher, climbed the redwood tree in his backyard and installed a lighted holiday sign that says HOPE. Now, in January 2009, the sign still hangs in the branches, swaying and sparkling all night.

It had an unexpected impact on our neighborhood. People from all over Berkeley came to gaze at the lights shifting in the wind. The *San Francisco Chronicle* even published an article about it, complete with photographs and interviews.

The HOPE sign inspired the theme for Paul and Bonnie's holiday poetry party in December. Guests brought poems with four words that started with the letters h, o, p, and e. Cooper's said, "Health enters our parents." My neighbor Margo read, with tears in her eyes, "Excruciating operation, peaceful healing."

I cling to hope while holding the possibility that I'm more likely near the end.

On a dull, winter day in early February, Tanya, Cooper, and I drive over the bridge to Marin County to see an oncologist who is said to be "open to alternatives." Arriving early, we stroll along a trail by the bay, gazing at Mount Tamalpais rising into a foggy, gray sky.

Dr. Gullion meets with us for an hour and a half. His assessment is not much different from what I'd heard from the surgeon at Stanford: I'm terminal. But Dr. Gullion stretches my time to possibly two years.

"Try chemotherapy," he says.

"Have you ever seen a miracle?" I finally ask.

"I've seen cancer disappear when we had no idea why. Go to Stanford and get their opinion, and we can decide from there."

He hugs me goodbye, and I'm startled to realize that I've never been hugged by a doctor through this entire ordeal!

We're glum on the drive home. The thought of pumping chemicals into my veins feels wrong. I know how bad the suggested protocol is. It would be worse than the chemotherapy I had for lymphoma twenty-three years ago, just after Cooper's birth. If I take it, I'll be in bed, feeling horrible for much longer than I was then. And if it can't cure me, why do it?

"Cooper, you can walk the dog or put your mother to bed," Tanya says after we get home.

"I'll put Marti to bed." It's not that I need to be "put to bed." It's just that I need a nap. A few minutes later, while I'm cleaning the kitchen, Cooper says, "I'll be upstairs, Mom."

When I come up, he's sitting in the chair by my bed with a game of Sudoku. I nestle under the comforter, and Cooper stays almost the whole time that I nap, enveloping me in love.

Reluctantly, I email my cancer list with the news that doctors think I am terminal, that I have several months to two years to live, that chemotherapy will not cure me, but it might buy more time.

Some decisions are easy, I write. I announce that I'm closing my business to spend as much time as possible with family and close friends. "While I maintain hope, I'm also realistic."

The only difficult decision is whether to bother getting chemotherapy at all.

A day later, Cooper, Tanya, and I go to Stanford to see what a second oncologist has to say. The prognosis isn't different: I'm terminal. But the options are interesting. Dr. Colevas recommends that I do nothing now. "Wait," he says, "and see what happens. The only concerns at the moment are the two very small nodules." If things progress, which he says is likely, the options will include four trials of experimental drugs and regimens that will have only minor side effects.

We leave Stanford with a sliver of hope.

As news of my diagnosis spreads, the weekend fills with lovely visits, walks and talks with my nearest and dearest. My friend Leann comes over with stories. She tells me about our mutual friend who has a fourteen-year-old son. He comes to her, a lesbian, and says, "Mom, you told me if I needed condoms, I should talk to you. I need them."

She gulps and goes to the pharmacy with her younger son, who's nine. After looking at the shelves of condoms without a *clue* which to choose, she talks to the pharmacist. "I'm a lesbian, I don't know anything about condoms, and I need some for my son."

The pharmacist looks down at her nine-year-old, who covers his crotch with both hands and yells, "Not for me!"

I'm laughing so hard that tears run down my face.

Later, I spend an hour and a half walking with Ann, which tells me how much life force I still have. "I can still see you sitting on the couch the first time we met," she says. "I loved you right away."

I recall that first meeting. It was 1975 at the War Resisters League office in San Francisco. David and I had driven down from Ukiah for an organizing meeting for the Continental Walk for Disarmament and Social Justice. Activists, peaceniks, and Buddhist monks were planning to walk from San Francisco to Washington, D.C. David and

I made a pitch for starting the walk in Ukiah, in rural America, and offered to organize the stretch from Ukiah to San Francisco. As was usual in those days, the room was filled with disheveled lefty men with long hair and scruffy beards. Ann and I were among only a handful of women in the room, and we became close friends over the course of the next year.

Today, we reminisce about the ups and downs of our friendship. "I remember there was a time we were angry with each other," I say, "but I can't remember why."

"I think I abandoned you when you had cancer the first time," she says. "It was totally unconscious. I just couldn't cope with losing you after losing Linda." Linda was Ann's sister who died in a car accident when Ann was seventeen, following the death of her father when she was twelve. As an adult, she's worked mightily to come to terms with these losses: working in therapy, volunteering at hospice, getting advanced degrees in gerontology and social work, reading and reading and reading, starting the world's first Grief Camp. She's an expert in grief.

"How's this going to be for you?" I ask.

"Right now it feels like lead in my veins. I haven't cried. I've just talked to the rabbi at work and to John." She met John, her husband, while doing hospice work.

"Please don't be strong for me," I say.

"I couldn't," she says. "You know I can't hide anything from you."

By Sunday afternoon, it's pouring rain, but I'm cozy in my friend Mary's dining room, drinking tea and talking. She asks how I am, and I get teary. "The tears come whenever they want to. It's amazing. I'm not this way. My brain has stopped monitoring everything. The feelings just rise up and come out. I cry when I'm happy. I cry when I'm sad. And what's weird is that I feel joy so much of the time."

—

My sixtieth birthday arrives in the midst of coming to grips with my terminal diagnosis. I've been psychologically preparing for it since I was fifty-eight and decide not to have a party. After all, we had our big wedding just five months ago. I don't need another celebration. Tuesday feels like any other day, except there are more flowers. Zillions of them. Daffodils from my neighbor Renate. An abundant arrangement of daffodils and iris from a group of women mediators I have met with for the past seventeen years. An azalea from my neighbors Sondra and Paul. Forsythia, yellow and vibrant, from my mother. An ikebana arrangement from our friend Nancy. Roses from Ann and John.

Tulips from Pam and Steve. I met Pam the first night of law school. She walked across the room with her halo of blond curly hair and introduced herself. We joined the same study group, prepared for the bar exam together, and have been close friends for almost forty years.

I told Cooper not to get me a present. "I don't need anything," I said. He surprises me with a card. "I'm so grateful," it says, "to have been given the last twenty-two years to spend with you. Every day I'm lucky to have you in my life. You've been a great mother and there isn't anything that you could have done differently. All in all, I think everything turned out pretty good. You've given me so much support and loads of opportunity so that I may prosper. You are amazing! I love you so much!"

I hug him fiercely.

The day after my birthday, I return to the medical grind for an appointment with Gabriella, my "integrative medicine" doctor and an old friend we met at Camp It Up, a family camp for "lesbian and gay families and their friends." We started going to it in 1990, when Cooper was four years old, so he'd see other families that looked like ours. We slept on hard mattresses on the floor of tent cabins in the northern California woods. It was hot, dusty, dirty, fun, exhausting, nourishing. It wasn't until Cooper was thirteen that he realized what our camp was about. "Have you ever noticed that there are a lot of lesbians at this camp?" he asked.

I'd called Gabriella recently to ask her if she'd be my primary care physician because I need help coordinating my care. I've been overwhelmed trying to manage all my treatments, which range from Western medicine to many alternative remedies. A friend and an MD, as well as a homeopath and an acupuncturist, Gabriella felt like just the right person to guide me.

Today, we spend an hour talking about my life and my temperament so that she can figure out my "constitutional remedy." In homeopathy, if you get this remedy right, they say, miracles happen. She asks more probing questions than a therapist, trying to find out what's unique about me. We talk about things we've never talked about before. My father: Navy captain; Southern gentleman; both tender and removed; at sea a lot when I was a kid; a quiet, go-to-sleep-early alcoholic who stopped drinking in his late fifties after my mother left him for six months while he sobered up. My mother: A Texan; a whirlwind; at the center of everything; life of the party; a talker. My ex-husband: Safe, controlling, and almost twenty years older than me. Tanya: a doer, not a talker; funny; full of energy; exuberant. My ambivalence about what I want, a long-term habit, my unconscious mantra carried over from childhood: Why figure out what you want when you won't get it anyway?

With this information in hand, Gabriella will figure out my remedy.

"What about Valentine's Day?" I ask. Cooper, Tanya and I are hanging out, talking about this and that. He says he's getting a telephone headset for Hayley.

"You gotta get something *romantic* for Valentine's Day," Tanya and I say in unison.

"This *is* romantic."

"How so?"

"Because when she gets off work at night and she's driving home, she's scared to talk very long on the cell phone. With the headset, we can talk the whole drive home if we want to."

"You better get a card and explain why you think it's romantic," I say. "And get some chocolate to go with it. You know she loves dark chocolate."

"Here's what I think is romantic," he says. "I'm going to get reservations at Point Reyes. There's nothing more romantic than putting your sleeping bags together and snuggling." A great idea except when it's February and freezing cold and raining, but I refrain from giving him more advice. I keep having to remind myself that he gets to run his own life.

Just after Valentine's Day, our neighbor Lonnie calls. She's the adult daughter of our long-time neighbor Reggie, who's in his nineties.

"I don't know about your faith," Lonnie, a devout Catholic, says, "but I have some blessed water from Lourdes. If you'd like some, I'd like you to have it. My father and I will bring it to you."

"No need. I'll come there," I say. "It's pouring rain. It's easier for me to come to you."

I dash down the street to their house, chat a while, and then Lonnie gives me a little wooden bottle with the holy water in it. Back home, I put it on our mantle above the fire, while I consider when to use it.

Later, I talk by phone to both of my brothers. As children, we had to rely heavily on each other, since we moved every year or two and had to start all over with new friends after each move. As the only girl, and the oldest, I was, in some ways, less connected to each of them than they were to each other. But we were close, off and on, during most of our lives.

Whit, two and a half years younger than I am, now lives in Boulder with his wife, Mary, and their son Martin, who carries on the family name. Whit is an acupuncturist and a teacher of acupuncture. He's also in great pain, due to a back injury, so we talk about *his* health for a while instead of *mine*, a welcome relief. Now that I've suffered chronic pain from my neck surgeries, I cannot imagine how he's managed over two years of it. He's on the verge of submitting to back surgery, something he's valiantly tried to avoid.

He tells me that Warren, my other brother, who's almost five years younger than I am, wants to visit me. Battling addiction since he was a teenager, Warren has been a merchant marine, a nurse, and now, who knows? He's clean and sober and looking for work in Hawaii, where he just moved from Hood River, Oregon.

"This is a really bad time," I say, almost panicked. "I'm closing my business and it takes absolutely all of my energy. I don't have the qi for a visit until that's done."

"Then you have to tell him that," Whit says.

I call Warren. "This may sound morbid," he says, "but if I could change places with you, I would. I don't have a partner or a child. If I died now, I'd be okay with it."

I'm a little surprised. "It doesn't work that way, does it?"

"No, but I'm praying every day."

"If prayers work," I say, "I should get a miracle. There are lots of people praying for my health."

"They work," he says. "But I don't pray for specifics. I just pray for you. Who knows what's supposed to happen?"

Managing my mind has become a major project. It bounces from thoughts and feelings like the little ball that bounced from word to word on the TV screen when I was a kid. When fear arises, it begins in my guts. It's fluttery, almost like excitement, but not quite. Perhaps it's more like anxiety. Then, my mind latches on to thoughts and races to the past or the future, anywhere but now. I'm learning to breathe through it and focus on the present, and the fear usually doesn't last very long.

Each night just before bed, I meditate. My friend Billie brought me a Medicine Buddha postcard that was blessed by her spiritual teacher. She says Tibetan monks all around the world are chanting for me. I light a candle, gaze at the card, and sit quietly, following my breath. At the end of my meditation, I'm always calm.

I'm learning to live with both hope and fear.

CATAPULTING INTO THERAPY

My first lesbian relationship doesn't last long, just one short month, from December 1980 into January, at which point Tanya decides to try to work things out with Betsy. I'm both disappointed and relieved. It turns out that having an open marriage was not so simple, at least for David and me. Our marriage has been shaken to the core; we're both reeling from the effects of my month-long relationship. David is hurt and lonely, not at all like Harold Nicholson. And I'm no Vita. Being intimate with two people at one time was excruciating.

"This was a *horrible* mistake," I say to David. "I'm so sorry I've hurt you."

"We were crazy to think this would work," he says. "It sounded good on paper, but the last month has been awful."

We make a pact not to rock the boat—no more open marriage. The plan is to get me through my last semester of law school and the bar exam and then, in August, to sort it all out with a good therapist.

Five months later in May, I'm sound asleep on a Saturday morning in my flat in San Francisco. It's my very last week of law school and I'm supposed to drive up to Ukiah today because David is baptizing his first grandchild, the son of his son "Little" David. I'm anxious about the trip because I'm uncomfortable that David's son is having a child before I do. It's not the right order, and there's still tension between David and me that we've never worked out about whether we'll even have a child together. My ambivalence, coupled with his reluctance, has resulted in no decision, even though at several points I've wanted to become pregnant.

My phone rings, waking me up early, before my alarm goes off.

"I just wanted to tell you that I slept with Joan last night," David says. All I know about Joan is that she's one of David's new Christian friends who had been present at the home birth of his grandson. "But I still want you to be at the baptism. She'll be there, too, and I'd like her to be able to come to the reception afterward."

I feel slapped. He's so calm, as if he hasn't just seriously jeopardized our fragile stability. "This has nothing to do with our relationship," he says flatly. "I was just taking care of myself."

"This wasn't our *agreement!*" I shriek into the phone. I can't believe he thinks I'll come to the baptism and smile at Joan.

I call my friend Ann to get her to drive with me to Ukiah. I need her support. We arrive while David's at church and gather all the things I think I'll need for a while: clothes, books, jewelry. I note with contempt that he slept with Joan in *our* bed. I leave Ukiah before David returns to our home.

This incident becomes the first time in our marriage that David and I aren't able to talk things through. We talk on the phone over the next week and every call ends with no resolution. I feel like I can't connect with him at all. He's unwilling to see that his actions do impact our marriage. He's unapologetic. We catapult into therapy with a psychiatrist in San Francisco recommended by his best friend, despite my serious need to focus on the bar exam.

David drives down from Ukiah for our first session, which is a few weeks after his night with Joan. After brief preliminaries, the therapist says, "I want you to play a game. Are you willing?"

"Sure," I say.

David hesitates, then agrees.

Jane gives us each a foam sword. "Fight," she says.

We stand up, feeling awkward, and start swinging. After a while, I begin to wail away at David, yelling furiously. David, who's six-four to my five-six, fights back, but he looks like a wimp to me.

"Stop!" Jane yells. She motions us to sit. "What did you see?"

I wait to see what David will say, but he's silent. Naturally, I think. He's so withholding.

Finally I say, "I was fighting David, and he wasn't doing much to fight back. He mostly defended himself." I sit up straight, proud of my insight.

"Do you want to know what I saw?" she asks, looking at me intently. I nod, a bit unsure. "I saw you making a lot of noise and being totally ineffective. David was in control the entire time. You accomplished nothing."

I'm speechless.

She turns to David, leans forward, and pummels him with questions, like a lawyer during cross-examination. "What do you want from Marti? How's this going to work?" Finally, after forty minutes of staccato question and answer, she summarizes, "So, you want Marti to finish law school, come back to Ukiah, and live happily ever after with you behind a white picket fence. She'll come to church on Sundays, sit in the front pew, and you'll be in control. She'll be a dutiful daughter and you'll be a benevolent father."

"Yeah, I guess that's right," he admits, reluctantly.

At that *precise* moment, time is up.

On the way out of her office, David says, "I can understand why you would want to be divorced from me, but I still want to be with you."

I'm mute. In shock. It's as if the veil has been lifted and I can see clearly for the first time.

Fortunately, a few hours later, David has to return to Ukiah to prepare for Sunday services, and I don't have to interact with him more at this moment.

I need time alone to process what's happening.

The next afternoon, I leave my flat in San Francisco and drive down to the hills above Redwood City, where I'm studying for the bar exam with my friend Pam. I've rented a little cottage next to her house that her landlord is letting me use Sunday night through Friday afternoon. On weekends, I return to my flat in San Francisco.

After sunset, I stand on the hill and look down at the lights of the Peninsula and the darkness of the Bay. In the distance, a strip of lights snakes along the East Bay hills on the horizon. The moonless sky is enormous, filled with stars. A light, warm breeze rises from the flatlands.

This thought bubbles up: "I want a divorce."

And that's it. I feel clear, light, exhilarated, without a shred of ambivalence.

Later that same evening, Pam comes out to my cottage. "Tanya's on the phone," she says. I'm bewildered that she's calling; we haven't seen or spoken to each other in six months.

"I've split up with Betsy," she says. "Are you available?"

I'm awed by the timing.

"Yes."

MOMENT TO MOMENT

In late February 2009, as I follow Dr. Colevas's advice to do nothing and see what happens, I notice a funny little protrusion along the scar line on my neck. Leaning into the mirror, I run my fingers against it. It's soft, flesh-toned, not at all like the two cancerous areas we already know about. My stomach tightens, but my mind wants to say it's nothing.

That afternoon Tanya notices. "What's this on your neck?"

"It's nothing," I insist.

"I think we should report this to the doctor. He said to report any changes."

"Okay, tomorrow morning. It's too late today."

The next morning, I call Stanford and talk to Jamie, one of the nurses who works with Dr. Colevas. I describe the blip. She tells me that she'll talk to the doctor and get back to me.

Then Tanya and I go to therapy. In the car, my tears rise and overflow. I'm afraid. "I just wanted one more week like last week, with no medical appointments and a little space to relax."

In therapy, we talk about having joy despite all the physical issues. "Last week, you were facing all this cancer business," our therapist says, "and you still had a wonderful week. What made it so great?"

"Going moment by moment," I say. "Very few plans. No medical appointments. Figuring out what we wanted to do as we went along through the day."

We emerge into the bright sun on Solano Avenue, the first sun in over a week of heavy, gray fog. At home, we walk Mollie around the block, take her back home, and stroll all the way back to Solano to take ourselves out to lunch. Then, we nap, blanketed in the late afternoon sun.

Our neighbor Joe sends an email asking if people want him to take down the HOPE sign.

I respond: "I really love the HOPE lights, and since hope is a big part of my psyche right now, it's nice to see the lights up there when we walk at night."

Joe writes: "A poet friend of mine, when she heard about the lights, wrote me that the tree itself is the light. She's right, but not completely right. I think that you are the light. At least you are one of my inspirations."

My health insurance bill for February arrives. Last month it was a whopping $867, *just for me*. The new bill is absurd: $1,128 per month, just for me. I want to scream when I realize that this new rate is my sixtieth birthday present.

I've just computed my out-of-pocket medical expenses for 2008, which were over $20,000, not including my health insurance, an additional $10,000. All in a year that I barely worked and had to put savings into my business to keep it "open." I remind myself that I'm "lucky" to have both health insurance and private disability insurance to see me through times like this, and that I could be suffering a lot more. We could have been financially devastated as a result of my cancer. I know that I'm fortunate that we paid premiums for over thirty years to protect us at times like this. But right now, at this particular

moment, I don't feel lucky. I just feel enraged about our dysfunctional health care system.

A lot of my social connections revolve around small groups: my girls'
club, my writing groups, my so-called book club. A meeting of that
book club is a sweet diversion from cancer. We began as a group of
women lawyers, therapists, and mediators intending to read books
about mediation and family law. That lasted about three months,
because the truth is we didn't want to be so academic. Then, we decided
to read fiction, which has been more successful. And now, we seem to
have morphed into a social club to which we bring our spouses for
dinner and conversation. We're now a group of three lesbian couples
and one heterosexual couple. We call Alan our honorary lesbian.

"What's it like being retired?" Mary asks Alan, who recently
stopped working.

"When you live your life always *doing* things, it's weird to wake up
and have the day unfold."

I like this image of the day unfolding, days where almost nothing
is scheduled, so that deciding what to do can actually be a moment-
by-moment experience. I think about my professional life of To Do
lists and have no desire to return to it.

"How is it closing your practice?" someone asks me.

"The decision was easy, but if I get my miracle, I'll have to figure
something else out. What's weird is that I'm not worried about it. I
just know that I can't return to sitting between two people who are
fighting. It makes my body cringe. I can't do it anymore."

I'm surprised that I don't feel any grief about giving up my business. All I feel is relief every time I delete an email about continuing
education, conferences, meetings, and rule changes.

—

Late on a Sunday night in February, I climb the stairs so exhausted that tears are gushing down my face. I've just spent an hour with Cooper working on his résumé, which he needs for his job search. His six-month water conservation job ended in December and he's busy looking for something meaningful. Many of his fellow graduates are working as baristas. He hopes he won't have to do that.

I knew I was exhausted and shouldn't be working late. The weekend was too busy. People came to visit. Some stayed *way* too long. I sat there dumbly, numbly, conversing and smiling, the ever-polite Southern hospitality oozing from me, inspired by my mother and grandmother, while inside all I wanted was to climb into bed and read and rest and be alone.

What is this need I have to take care of others at my own expense?

When I get to bed, I find Tanya, who has sensibly gone to bed already. She wakes up when she hears me sniffling and wraps her arms around me until I fall asleep.

The next morning, I groan as I turn the page of my calendar to a new week. It's filled with medical appointments all over the Bay Area, from Stanford to Novato. Fortunately, today's appointment is the most interesting. One of my favorite clients sent me a card when I notified her that I was closing my practice. She wrote about a healer she'd been to after a breast cancer scare. I checked out his website and decided to go see him. Why not? What do I have to lose?

Tanya and I drive up to Novato, where his house sits on the top of a hill, looking out over vibrant green hills dotted with oak and madrone. We walk down a path on the side of the house into a long, narrow office with windows overlooking a canyon. The healer emerges from a back room to greet me, his face startlingly beautiful and serene, his gaze direct. In his office, he asks a number of questions about my condition and suggests a few alternative treatments to consider.

"I'd like to do some hands-on work. May I touch you?" he asks. I appreciate that he asks for permission.

"Yes." I climb onto his massage table, fully clothed.

He begins to work to deepen and slow my breathing. He murmurs quietly into my ear, softly touches my neck, head, chest, diaphragm.

"The way to eliminate cancer is not to fight it and not to focus on it," he says. "Focus on *living*. Imagine yourself in 2021, healthy and vibrant. Don't spend all your time talking to people about the cancer."

Time passes. I feel like I'm floating, and when the session is over, I'm utterly calm.

On Tuesday, I return to the valley of the shadow of death, the Stanford Cancer Center, for another PET scan. Three hours of driving, one and a half hours of testing, and then the long wait until Friday to get the results.

On Wednesday, I see my *last* couple with an active mediation. They've stayed with me for the fourteen months since my diagnosis, accommodating my off-again, on-again schedule. As I greet them at my front door, I wonder how I'll feel when they leave.

It's clear almost immediately that we won't be able to finish their divorce agreement. They still need to have a detailed and thoughtful conversation about spousal support. I feel the tug in me. I know exactly how to structure this discussion. I know what they need to do and how to help them do it. But I also know I *have* to stop.

I breathe deeply, and say, "The two of you need to have a discussion about spousal support. I don't think it's something we can rush through and I'm not going to be able to do this with you."

They look at me across the table. "We know, Martina. You have to take care of yourself." They are so generous and kind, I get teary. I give them the name of a colleague and friend, and tell them I will help in the transition.

We spend the rest of our time together talking about the economy, their work (art), their spiritual practice (Buddhist), shamanic practices of healing. When they leave, I don't charge them and we hug each other goodbye. I close the front door and walk into the living room feeling light, unburdened, and ready for whatever comes next.

On Friday of my jam-packed week, Tanya and I drive to Stanford to see my oncologist for the results of the scan. My appointment time is 1:30 p.m., but Dr. Colevas doesn't appear until 4:00! He had an emergency early in the morning and was behind all day. I've read most of the two *New Yorkers* I brought and am about to finish *The Week* when he comes into the examining room in his signature bowtie. He's sincerely apologetic.

The usual poking, prodding, and fingers down my throat ensues before we get the test results. The PET scan shows the two nodules on my skin that we already knew about, and one more, farther inside, which is still small. I'm actually somewhat relieved by the results, as I was worried there was a bigger tumor that was the cause of the "blip" along the incision.

Dr. Colevas suggests a chemotherapy regime that is not super-toxic, or further "close monitoring." My choice.

"I'll think about it over the weekend," I say.

"I'm going to set things up for you to start," Dr. Colevas says. "It's easier to cancel chemo than to start it."

"Okay," I say. "I'll let you know what I decide."

Tanya and I race home in rush-hour traffic for a date with Cooper and Hayley at O Chame for his twenty-third birthday. Our reservation is for 6 p.m. When we arrive at 6:15, the two of them are cuddled in a booth waiting for us. We munch on onion pancakes, grilled eel on endive, blanched spinach with sesame/miso sauce, and thin slices of flank steak, followed by caramel balsamic gelato with a candle.

LOBBING GRENADES

I've just spent another weekend with David in San Francisco. It's the weekend after I told him I wanted a divorce. He's hurt, angry, impossible to talk to. My previously kind and gentle husband has become a lunatic! In the past week, he's taken my name off all our bank accounts. He's cut me off medical insurance, knowing how hard it will be to get insurance with no job and preexisting conditions related to a series of abnormal pap smears. Even though I've graduated from law school, I'm studying for the bar exam and have no earnings yet. When I confront him about the health insurance, he says, "I can't have the church paying your medical insurance when we're getting a divorce." He's so self-righteous!

I'm well aware that I could get the divorce court to order him to maintain my health insurance and even pay me spousal support. But I don't want his help. Instead, I get him to agree to reinstate my insurance if I pay for it.

The entire weekend has been excruciating, and I'm relieved to be dropping him off at the Greyhound station for his trip back to Ukiah.

"Oh, by the way, your mother called me this week," he says as he gets out of the car.

He closes the car door, leans in the window, and casually says, "She asked me if homosexuality had anything to do with our divorce. I told her about you and Tanya."

I'm aghast.

He turns on his heel and is on his way to Ukiah to preach.

It's not like I was planning to come out to my family right now. The divorce is enough for all of us to absorb. It's true, I've begun to see Tanya. And yes, it's likely I'll be with women if I'm not with David. But it's not like I feel ready to make an *announcement*.

And it's not like we landed in therapy because *I* wanted to leave the marriage. It was *his* affair that broke our agreement to end our experiment with open marriage, and, of course, he failed to mention his affair to my mother. What a hypocrite.

That night, I call San Diego and speak with my mother. I tell her the whole story, not just my part of it. I can tell she's upset. She and David are close. My parents know Tanya from when we worked together. But, of course, that was when neither of us thought we were anything but friends.

Reluctantly, I ask if I can borrow $3,000 from her and my father to get me through the bar exam. I tell her I don't want to spend my time fighting with David. She agrees to the loan.

In the next few weeks, David refuses my request to go to mediation to work out our divorce. Instead, he hires a mutual friend to be his lawyer and tells me that if I have something to say, I should have my lawyer call his lawyer.

He won't talk to me about a single thing.

After this conversation with my mother, I still have more work to do with my family. My brother Whit is in Beijing, studying acupuncture. There's no way to talk to him by telephone, so I write him a long letter about getting the divorce and seeing Tanya. His reply is full of his upset about all the ways that my divorce is wrecking *his* life! Which is true, in certain respects, since he's a part owner of the land where David and I live. Whit has a small yurt there, where he stays when he's in Ukiah. He considers our land his home, even though he's lived in LA and Beijing for a number of years while studying acupuncture. Without discussing it, we both know that we can't afford to buy David's interest and that the land will have to be sold.

Still, his anger stings.

I call my other brother, Warren, on the telephone. He's matter-of-fact and completely nonjudgmental about my divorce and unplanned coming out. "I always wondered whether David was right for you," is all he says. He and Tanya resonated the moment they met, and I can tell he already likes her.

My mother is sad about the divorce. She comes to San Francisco from San Diego to visit for a few days. "Won't you miss a penis?" she asks as we stroll arm in arm down Irving Street. I can't *believe* my mother is asking me this question and laugh out loud.

"Lesbians are quite inventive," is all I'll say. I avoid Tanya while my mother's in town, feeling she won't welcome Tanya yet.

Frankly, I have no memory of talking to my father about any of my monumental life changes. But years later, I'll learn that he cried when he heard the news: not about David, whom he didn't like much, but about my being a lesbian. But this initial reaction doesn't keep him from coming to adore Tanya within a few years.

Meanwhile, Tanya and I begin our Lesbian High Drama stage. My experiment with David has taught me that I'm not interested in multiple partners. I can't manage this free-to-be-you-and-me lifestyle, even though it sounds great in principle and would make life infinitely easier, given the times.

But Tanya's like a person who's been let out of prison. She loves me, but she's not remotely interested in monogamous commitment.

We get together. We split up. We get back together. We split up.

Finally, I call it off. I date other women. I move on. I finish my excruciating divorce. I go to therapy. I cry a lot. I learn to be a lawyer, to bill hours, to dress like a professional, to save money.

When I finally complete my divorce in 1982, I'm thirty-three years old and have never lived alone. I move into a tiny Berkeley attic apartment, all by myself. I walk up the long flight of stairs into one big room surrounded with little windows looking out onto treetops. A cozy tree house, except it needs attention.

Finally, I get my meager settlement from David—there really wasn't much to fight about. I pay my lawyer and my parents and have just enough left to carpet my studio and have the walls painted. I move in my overstuffed couch that I got from Maggie when she left Ukiah for chiropractic school, buy a bed, hang my art on the walls, and settle into my little nest.

After six months, I hear through mutual friends that Tanya is not doing well. She's depressed, in therapy, not seeing anyone, blaming herself for wrecking our relationship. I figure I should let her off the hook, let her know that I understand how hard it was to be with me. I've just stopped dating a woman who's a law student, and now I see how the dynamic works: the dependency, the lack of money, the neediness, the anxiety. I finally get it that I was hardly a catch when I was finishing law school, in debt, studying for the bar exam, starting a new job, getting a divorce, and coming out. I figure I might as well tell her that it wasn't *all* her fault! The last time we'd split up, I'd been a self-righteous nutcase.

I invite her to dinner in my little studio. On the night she's coming, I tidy up and make brown rice, tofu, and veggies, because I'm still a hippie at heart.

Tanya trudges up the long staircase to my attic apartment. We haven't seen each other for months and talk long into the evening.

Nobody will believe me later when I say I had absolutely no

intention of getting back together with her, but get together we do. Given our LHD history, we don't tell *anyone*, not even our best friends, for three months. It takes us that long to trust that it's real this time, before we let ourselves sink into the arms of our relationship. And it takes even longer before we move in together into our little house on Albany Hill, where we live until Cooper is born.

DIFFICULT DECISIONS

I'm in turmoil. I can't decide whether to start chemo and I'm supposed to let Dr. Colevas know my decision. I keep wondering why I'd do it if it won't cure me. But somehow, saying no to chemo feels like giving up. The spot on my neck nags me: It's impossible to ignore. Every time I look in the mirror, it stares at me, inflamed and angry.

I decide to wait and see how I feel just before my next appointment in two weeks.

Then the blip on my neck opens up and oozes a little clear liquid and blood. How can I be hopeful when I can see the tumors every day? Even if I avoid looking, I still *feel* them. I always know they're there.

I made the decision to close my business in January, and although I've had my last in-person meeting with clients, the work of closing my practice is far from over. Doing so in a responsible way has been considerably more time-consuming that I expected. Now in mid-March, Kim is still working with me to finish the job. I'm so thrilled to move through this work that I'm focused all morning, although I know I'll pay the price for this effort tomorrow and the next day, when I'll be in bed with exhaustion.

Kim has worked for us so long that she's become part of the family. Before the economy crashed, getting a new job would have been a cinch for her, but now law firms are laying off both lawyers and legal secretaries and she's not even getting interviews. I'm worried; I want her settled in a new job when we're done with my work.

And we're almost done. I can feel it. I need the right spot to appear for Kim.

After she leaves, the house is totally quiet until I hear the mail plop onto the floor by the front door. I shuffle through bills and ads and find a letter announcing that I have been selected as a 2009 Super Lawyer. I stare at my name on the list and laugh out loud.

Tanya and I are gabbing in the living room late in the evening after a West Coast swing class when Cooper comes in from his cottage. Kim is not the only one having trouble finding a job. I lament that Cooper graduated from college just as the economy crashed.

"Let's go on a trip together to the river," he says. He's talking about our cabin on the Russian River, which, unfortunately, hasn't sold, also because of the economy.

It's been a long time since Cooper has wanted to vacation with us. What will he do with no TV, no Internet, nothing happening except the rushing river and a lot of serenity?

But on Saturday morning, he's ready to go at ten. We load up, stop in Graton for lunch, and get to our cold, damp cabin on aptly-named Freezeout Road in the early afternoon.

The ritual of arrival: Haul wood. Start a fire. Put away supplies. Settle in. When it finally warms up, we play games—Jenga and Sequence—and lounge around reading and blabbing.

"Let's go tide-pooling," he says as he checks his tide book. "It's low tide late tomorrow afternoon. I'll take you to Shell Beach."

The next afternoon, we hike down many stairs to a beach on the Sonoma coast where it's so windy that I have to brace myself to keep from being blown over. The air is crisp, the water shimmering, the waves frothy, the tide pools teeming with starfish, anemones, mussels, seaweed of all colors. We hop over boulders, collect rocks, breathe the salt air. Finally, hiking back up all the stairs to the car, I find I'm not out of breath. I love feeling strong and healthy.

But on the way home the next day, I fall back into an abyss of fear, just like that. We stop on the way for an appointment with another healer recommended by a close friend. I meet with her for two hours and take fifteen pages of notes that say things like: Do coffee enemas four times a day; don't do chemotherapy; drink native American tea; wash veggies in distilled water, not tap water; eat plankton; drink chlorophyll water; eat only organic fruits and veggies and grains from her list.

"This is all-out war," she says.

That night, I wake up in the middle of the night gripped by fear, stomach gnawing, heart fluttering, muscles tense. I breathe. I visualize. I meditate. I do everything I know how to do, but I am unable to calm down. Hope is out of reach.

After a second night of wrenching fear, I wake up sobbing. "I'm not brave enough to refuse chemotherapy."

Tanya simply holds me. I know she doesn't have an agenda about what I should do. Or, if she does, she hides it well. It's a relief not to have pressure from her. The first time I had cancer, she said she got to vote for herself and Cooper to override any decisions I made that worried her. Usually Miss Fix-It, she's figured out from the cancer this time that there's absolutely nothing she can do. She's read many books, currently *The Tibetan Book of Living and Dying*, and has absorbed the lessons well. All day long, off and on, I'm in tears. All she does is love me and hug me and tell me she'll be here with me, whatever I decide.

"My job is to take in your fear and reflect back love and compassion," she says, quoting from her reading. These are definitely not words she'd use! This is a woman who was raised in Texas by

Southern Baptists. She hated it, but toed the line. Her summers were spent in vacation bible school and at big-tent revivals led by relatives. Being baptized meant that you were dunked in water, full body. As an adult, she's not been spiritually inclined. In our twenty-eight years together, she's never done anything overtly spiritual except play gospel music on the piano. But she supported me in meditating and going on retreats. She supported Cooper in his coming-of-age process with the Berkeley Zen Center. She's just never been involved herself.

Now she's like a bodhisattva, shining her love on me every moment I'm around her.

In the middle of the terrors on the third night, I realize that I've been hijacked by all my old psychological garbage: I'm doing something wrong. This must be my fault. I'm not good enough. Not pure enough. Not perfect enough. Not working hard enough to get over this.

Such old, old messages, hardwired deep inside, waiting to be triggered.

I make a decision about the alternative treatments suggested by the healer three days ago. Any miracle cure will be just that—a miracle on a spiritual level, mostly out of my control and certainly not the result of four enemas a day and concentration on therapies 24/7.

I go back to sleep and when I wake up, I'm myself again.

Meanwhile, I continue to see the Novato healer. He's referred to as Master by the people who work with him, and though I respect him immensely, I can't bring myself to call him that. I call him Healing Man. He's given me instructions to train my mind, to say, "STOP" when it dwells on cancer. "Say it quietly, but firmly. Sizzle those negative thoughts out."

In spite of my years of meditation practice—albeit sloppy, sporadic, neglected for months at a time—I'm shocked by how undisciplined my mind is. It goes wherever it wants to, and too often it goes to worry.

"Worry mind. STOP," I say gently.

After several weeks of this practice, I see that I'm calmer. I feel better. My mind still does the same thing, but less often and less intensely. When I talk firmly, but kindly, to worry mind, worry mind stops.

I walk in the front door after a luxurious spa date with Ann. I'm relaxed. Radiant. Happy. Cooper's on the couch.

"How'd it go?"

"I fucked up, Mom." The look on his face tells me otherwise. He's grinning.

He's just had an interview at Marin Water District. He gives me the blow-by-blow, and it sounds like he did just fine, but he's such a perfectionist that anything short of great is a problem in his view.

I think about how it was for me at his age. When I left Pomona College in 1969 and moved to San Francisco, I had a job in twenty-four hours and soon thereafter, a flat with Cindy at 18th and Sanchez that cost us $300 a month. My $500 paycheck paid my share of the rent, food, clothing, Muni fares, entertainment, and I *still* had money left over.

And here's Cooper, infinitely more qualified than I was then, living in the garage apartment behind our house, wondering how long it will take to land the next job.

In mid-March, I have my appointment at Stanford. Up at 5:00 a.m. In the car at 5:45. Arrive at Stanford at 7:00. Oatmeal and fresh fruit. Blood draw at 7:30. Dr. Colevas at 8:00. I think I'm going to have chemotherapy at 8:30, because I never called to cancel it. I was simply too indecisive. Talk about passively backing your way into a medical decision!

But after checking me out, Dr. Colevas decides not to proceed— at least not yet. I'm elated. Another appointment two weeks out. Another two weeks to magically melt my tumors away.

The next day, a letter addressed to Cooper Reaves drops through the mail slot. The return address says: Marin Water District. My stomach flips. I try to see through the envelope to see if he's been called back for a second interview. It's all I can do to refrain from tearing it open.

I call him, and when he finally pulls out the letter, he holds his breath. I look over his shoulder and see the bold type with the date and time of the next interview. He's in the top three. I'm ecstatic. It takes him awhile to digest the news, and then he slowly breathes again.

On a glorious spring day that vibrates with new growth and blazing sunlight, Ann and I walk up Oxford Street from Temple Beth-El, where she works as the interim director. I tell her about my packed week ahead.

"You have to cancel things," she says. "Take care of yourself first."

It's obvious that I'm not good at this. I don't want to hurt people's feelings. Emails arrive. "Can I drop by and see you?" It's not that these are people I don't want to see. It's that there are too many of them. Socializing, except in very small doses, is depleting. Finding a way to say no is difficult.

I never had to face this kind of problem until later in life. If you move all the time, as I did most of my life, your friends are scattered all over the place. But I've been in my Berkeley house with Tanya since

1986 and in the Berkeley area since 1981. We have friends, colleagues, neighbors—people who are important, but too numerous to connect with personally right now. I seem incapable of finding balance.

Ann hangs in with me. "What works for you?"

"Small, peaceful. Not too many people."

We walk quietly for a moment. "I hate to tell you this," I say, "but I just can't handle the Seder this year." The thought of being with a large group of people for three hours is just too much.

Ann does a Seder almost every year. It's an important ritual for her for many reasons, including that it's the holiday when her sister died. I've been to every Seder for over twenty years except one, when I was out of town on vacation.

"That's okay. We'll just have you and Tanya and John and me," she says. I'm touched by this response, and grateful to be able to spend the evening with her and John.

My girls' club meets on Dana's houseboat at the end of a pier in Sausalito. Six of us have been meeting for a day every month or two since 1992. Other than our meetings, we don't see each other day-to-day very often, but the intimate continuity has been a source of support all this time. We've seen each other through divorces, marriages, troubles, good times, kid problems, kid successes, business problems, health problems, career changes. Our primary commitment is to be honest with each other.

It's a bright, vibrant day. Seagulls flitter around, squawking. We make a scrumptious lunch—lentil soup, salad, almonds, strawberries, bread. We each get forty-five minutes of complete attention from our friends to talk about whatever is important to us.

I look at Maude. "You said you were dealing with 'What is.' What did you mean by that?"

"I'm having trouble with your illness," she says. "I don't want you to have to deal with it. I know you don't want to talk about it a lot, but I have to be honest about it."

I breathe. "I'm just trying to do my life," I say. "Each day. I'm more than my cancer, and I don't want to spend my time dwelling on it. I already spend hours and hours each week seeing doctors and health practitioners. I know we need to talk about it sometimes, but you need to know that thinking about it more than I already have to is not what I want to do."

They want to know how they can help.

"Just being here with you helps," I say. In fact, hearing them talk about their lives rather than focusing on *my* life is helpful.

This is what I see on my calendar for March 25, 2009: 10:00 a.m. therapy with Tanya and Cooper; 11:30 a.m. acupuncture; 2:30 p.m. appointment with Jill, my body worker; 4:00 p.m. appointment with my doctor Gabriella. How ridiculous is this day?

"Get going with the chemo, if you're going to do it," Gabriella says emphatically. "You can decide *not* to do it at all, but if you're going to do it, *now's* the time, while you still have some energy and you're not completely depleted."

This advice is a blow, but it knocks me out of my state of ambivalence. I trust Gabriella. It's the first time she's told me what to do.

And I know she's right. It's time for chemo.

NOTHING CAN STEAL OUR JOY

We sit in Tanya's brown Mazda on Castro Street on a foggy May afternoon in 1985, quietly waiting for our appointment time. Nobody knows our plan except my therapist and the two of us.

"Can't we go up now?" I ask.

"No," Tanya says. "They were emphatic that we not arrive early."

I gaze out the car window. At this moment, in broad daylight, you'd never know that at night the Castro is a gay mecca teeming with well-groomed gay men in flannel shirts and tight jeans and disheveled lesbians in work shirts and baggy jeans. Right now it looks just like any other San Francisco neighborhood of shops, cafés, and businesses, including the Castro Theatre, the Elephant Walk bar, and the storefront that used to be Harvey Milk's camera shop.

Tanya has always wanted kids. I've known this about her from the time we first met at Jerry Berg's law office. After we moved in together, as she talked about children more often, I realized that I needed to grapple with my own feelings about becoming a parent.

David and I had gotten divorced before we ever resolved the issue of children. "If you're *sure* you want a child," he'd said more than once, "then we'll have one." But he already had four from his previous marriage and was clearly unenthusiastic.

For one brief moment during our marriage, I was 100 percent ready. We were with close friends who'd announced that they were trying to have a baby. As the evening wore on, I said I wanted to get pregnant, too, and my friends and I got excited talking about how great it would be if we both got pregnant at the same time.

But on the long drive back to our land, David said he felt the time wasn't right and I never brought it up again. After that there wasn't another moment when I felt 100 percent certain.

Unlike Tanya, I didn't fantasize about being a mother. As a child, I didn't even like playing with dolls. I still remember the surge of relief I felt at age seven after I complained to my mother that my friend was coming over with her doll. My mother said, "You don't have to play dolls if you don't want to. You can do other things."

Everybody played dolls in the fifties. Everybody *had* dolls and you'd have been weird if you didn't like dolls. I managed this dilemma by *collecting* dolls. Every time my Navy captain father returned from being at sea, he brought me a new doll. I displayed them on a shelf in my bedroom and at one point had a collection of fifty from all over the world.

When I realized how much Tanya wanted children, I hauled myself off to therapy to grapple with my fears. By then, I wanted to make a family, too. But now I was aware of my multitude of worries: Would our baby be healthy? Would I be a good mother? How would people react? Would my career as a family lawyer suffer? Would people stop referring cases to me? How would our families take it? Did I even *care* whether they approved? I wasn't worried about Tanya. I knew she would be fine. She wasn't full of worries.

Eventually, I accepted reality. There aren't any guarantees. I wouldn't be a *perfect* parent, but I'd be a *good* parent. True, I'd be taking a chance with my career. Some people would disapprove. So what? It was worth the risk. I no longer needed to be 100 percent certain.

Because I was almost five years older than Tanya, we decided I would have our first child and Tanya the second. But our path wasn't clear. None of our lesbian friends had children. No lesbian mom handbook existed.

We considered asking a friend to be our donor, but our straight friends had wives who weren't comfortable with their husbands becoming donors. Our gay friends were at risk of AIDS, even though we didn't have full understanding about it then. Our friends didn't begin to die until 1986. In 1985, sperm banks avoided gay donors but still provided fresh sperm to their clients. We were also concerned that if we knew our donor, we might have problems if he changed his mind and wanted to become an involved parent. The law on this point was not settled.

So we turned to a sperm bank. The Yellow Pages led us to one in Berkeley. The sleek waiting room was full of heterosexual couples who stared at us as if we were freaks. Two women wanting an insemination were a rarity in 1985.

I quietly asked the receptionist for information.

"Here's our list," she said in a voice loud with judgment. She obviously disapproved of us. Their spreadsheet had columns labeled height, weight, age, hair color, and religion. No detailed information was included. It felt too much like picking out nail polish or a bottle of wine. It was too impersonal for me.

Tanya and I slunk out and never returned.

We were clear about three things. First, we wanted the boundaries of our family to be defined from the start: Tanya, me, and our child. We didn't want our donor to be involved in raising our child in any way. Second, we wanted a donor our child could meet when he or she grew up, which eliminated all the donors who wanted to remain completely anonymous. Third, we wanted fresh sperm. The idea of frozen sperm sounded like making Minute Maid orange juice with a can plucked from the freezer. It just didn't feel right. And we thought I'd have a better chance of getting pregnant with fresh sperm.

Several months after our depressing sperm bank experience, we

heard about Sherrin Mills, a nurse practitioner who was just beginning to serve lesbians who wanted children.

After our last adventure, it was a relief to visit a lesbian-friendly
facility. Sherrin gave us four-page bios for each donor who was willing to donate fresh sperm, meaning that he would be on call to come
to the office to make a donation when I was ovulating. Sherrin had
personally interviewed each man. We appreciated this more personal
approach.

Tanya and I studied the bios carefully and made our top three
choices, focusing on personality. Good looks were not a priority; we
wanted a man who was kind, sensitive, warm.

"Which one would you pick?" we asked Sherrin's secretary.
Secretaries *always* know what's really going on. She looked at our top
three and pointed without hesitation.

"This one. He's a cross between Bob Dylan and Woody Allen and
a *very* sweet man."

We looked at his essay one last time: "Maternity, birth, raising
an infant to adulthood, watching one's own child form his or her
unique selfhood—this can be one of the most exquisite and powerful
experiences of a lifetime. I wish to help those people who for physical
or philosophic reasons have turned to this unconventional and alternative approach in order to have a child of their own."

We'd found our man.

So here we are, sitting in Tanya's Mazda, counting the minutes before
our insemination appointment. Sherrin doesn't want us to come
early because she doesn't want us to run into the donor, who will be
in the next room. I suddenly find myself laughing. "I feel like we're
in a California farce. Can't you picture it? The sperm donor runs up
the stairs, late. The nervous lesbian couple arrives early and bumps
into the donor on the stairway. The sperm donor hangs out in one

room with *Playboy*. The lesbians wait impatiently in the next room for delivery of the goods."

Tanya rolls her eyes.

At the appointed time, we pass no one on the stairs. Sherrin escorts us to an examining room, I remove my underwear, climb onto the examining table, and she inserts the sperm, with a cap to hold it in. We're done in ten minutes. We meet our friend Phyllis an hour later for dinner, so giddy that we have to tell her our news.

"You're already pregnant!" she proclaims, clapping her hands. "I know it!"

Before we confirm we're pregnant, Tanya and I fly to San Diego to see my parents. We're sitting around the dining room table in their sun-drenched house on Capistrano Street, where they moved when my father retired from the Navy.

"We have something to tell you," I say.

They look at me expectantly.

"I'm trying to get pregnant by artificial insemination."

"Wonderful," my mother says immediately. "I *knew* that's what you were going to say." My mother *always* believes she knows what her children are thinking and that whatever we do is wonderful.

My father, normally a quiet Southern gentleman, pounds the table and yells, "We're *not* going to have a bastard in our family!"

My therapy has prepared me for this response (more or less). I have a reply ready and feel grateful that I anticipated this reaction. Otherwise the moment would have been hard.

"Dad, we're not having a bastard," I say calmly. "Tanya and I are having a baby *together*. There will be *two* parents and it'll be fine. I love you and I think you'll be a wonderful grandfather. Just let me know when you're ready. Until then, I'm going to leave you alone."

Tanya and I retreat to our bedroom and return to the Bay Area the next day as planned. My father is gracious while we're there and hugs us both goodbye. I know he can't help himself. And I feel sure he'll come around, because he loves me and he's at heart a sweet man. In the end, it only takes a few months for him to adjust to the new reality.

Phyllis's prediction was right: Despite the lack of romantic ambiance, I'm pregnant on the first try!

Being pregnant is easy: No morning sickness. No complications.

The difficulty is work. I know that my business partner will be a problem, so I don't tell her I'm pregnant until the first trimester is over. Although she's a lesbian, she believes that lesbians shouldn't have children, a view that is ubiquitous in the lesbian community at the moment. When she made me a partner, I told her that Tanya and I were planning to have a baby. But I think she believed that I would relent and embrace the child-free, lucrative lesbian-lawyer lifestyle.

I want to protect my baby and myself from stress and bad vibes, but at three months, I know I have to inform her. When I reluctantly make the announcement, she's infuriated.

She thinks I should have told her immediately. She's upset that I'll need maternity leave, indignant because in the natural order of things, as the new lawyer, I should be holding down the fort while she vacations in Italy. When Tanya and I learn that we're having a boy, she says, "Boys need to be raised by fathers."

Our office seethes with reproach, and I can hardly wait to leave.

I work until the morning of February 28, 1986, when my water breaks. Later in the day, sweet Cooper is born. For medical reasons, I need a C-section, so my part is easy. Cooper arrives unscathed by a journey through the birth canal, with creamy skin, dark hair, a curl in the middle of his forehead, and perfect little fingers that peek out from the top of his blanket. He's crying when the doctor puts him in my arms. I whisper into his ear, "Everything will be okay," and he settles down. Our room at Alta Bates fills with friends and flowers, and we are completely enchanted.

Two days later, when we come home from the hospital with Cooper, our phone rings almost immediately. Tanya answers. I can tell by the twang in her voice that it's *her* father, calling from the Bible Belt in Texas. She hangs up quickly. Grinning.

"You want to know what he's calling about?" she asks. Now she's laughing.

I nod.

"He's calling to make sure that I don't think *I'm* going to have a bastard like *you* just did!" For a moment, I'm furious. It's more upsetting than my own father using the word bastard. Maybe it's easier being mad at Tanya's father, but somehow his timing is more egregious. How dare he call the very day we bring Cooper home from the hospital?

Then I look down. Here we are in our tiny house, so completely thrilled to have our beautiful baby snuggled in our arms that we both start laughing. Southern men!

Nothing can steal our joy.

LET IT BEGIN

Tanya and I leave for my appointment at Stanford in the very early morning. At the hospital's entrance, I bliss out walking through the country garden blooming with fruit trees and zillions of tulips, phlox, and daisies. The scent is heavenly. We eat oatmeal and fruit in the cafeteria, get a blood test, and when we see Dr. Colevas, we decide to start chemo. *Today! March 29, 2009.*

The nurse directs us to the infusion room, which is a ridiculous name, in my opinion. It makes it sound like I'll be enjoying some kind of gourmet delicacy instead of being bombarded with toxic chemicals. The room is filled with reclining chairs next to a huge window that looks out over a park.

"Choose a chair," Nurse Ratchet says. She doesn't even say hello or tell me her name.

It takes her two pokes to get a correct vein. Drip. Drip. Drip. Lots of saline solution to hydrate me. Three kinds of chemotherapy. It's not done until very late in the afternoon, in part because my nurse doesn't have the next bag of chemicals ready when each one runs out, so there's a long wait between infusions. But by some grace of the universe, Friday night rush hour is not a rush hour, and we speed home.

To bed early. Deep, deep sleep.

—

The next morning, I feel wonderful. I'm amazed. I have lots of energy, no nausea, little pain. Could it be the prednisone? The other medications? I feel optimistic, despite having zero odds for a cure. And I have a whole weekend before me with not one social obligation! All weekend, I'm enlivened and happy, without worries. Spring is exploding around me: wisteria, yellow roses, wild irises. Plump succulents sprout new growth; purple broccoli, dahlias, and lilies poke up through the soil.

I have a visit with Maggie, who's been my friend since the 1970s. We met during college in Ashland, but became close when we lived in Ukiah and later, the Bay Area. She's visiting California from her hometown of Kenosha, Wisconsin, where she's refurbishing an old Tudor house on Lake Michigan and figuring out the next phase of her life.

Being with her is familiar. We talk shorthand. We don't talk health, neither her Lyme disease nor my cancer. We talk books, old friends, her new life in the Midwest, our kids, politics. When she leaves, I'm filled up and tired, but happy tired.

Tanya and I decide to cut back on therapy for a while, mostly because I have too many appointments every week and I desperately need more space. Cooper will continue with his individual therapy and we have a final session with him. During this appointment, he talks about wanting to be connected, how he feels like he has to reach through a Jell-O-like substance before he can get close to anyone.

That evening, Cooper ensconces himself upstairs in front of our new TV, watching movies. I'm downstairs, reading peacefully. Tanya's at our dance class, which I can no longer go to because of my low energy. Cooper comes downstairs.

"I feel guilty," he says.

"Guilt is a wasted emotion," I say automatically.

"Yeah, but I could have been hanging out with you, and instead I'm stuck in front of the TV."

"Coop, we're all doing the best we can," I say gently.

He plops into the chair across from me.

"What's going on?" I ask.

"I'm sad and confused."

"I'm so sorry my being sick is affecting your life in such a big way." I tear up.

He looks at me a long time. Then he stands up. Hands hanging at his side, he motions me over. We hug and cry. Minutes go by. Finally, I go get Kleenex for both of us and we sit down again.

"I'm so tired of being scared," he says.

"Are you scared I'm dying?"

"No, I'm scared of love," he says. "I know there's nothing to be afraid of, but I just get scared."

"To put things in perspective, you've got to give yourself credit. You were just open and vulnerable and loving in a way most people don't do easily."

We sit, deeply connected, for a few more minutes before he goes back to the TV and I return to my book.

"Martina, get on the phone!" Tanya yells. "Cooper wants to talk to both of us."

Uh-oh, I think. *What's wrong?*

"Are you both there?" he asks.

"Yes."

"Guess what?" he says. *Just spit it out*, I want to say.

"Cooper, tell us," Tanya says calmly.

"I've got a job offer at the Contra Costa Water District!" Not Marin, where he'd gotten to the final interviews, but Contra Costa.

"Did you take it?" we ask.

"I told them I had to think about it overnight."

We're relieved. At least he won't have to join his buddies as a barista. Still, only Cooper would play hard to get in this economy!

A week after my first chemo treatment, I'm back at Stanford again. Dr. Colevas says that my tumors have shrunk and that the CT scan shows no hidden time bombs. Yes! I'm in the infusion room by midmorning.

As I choose my chair, I'm told that I'm assigned to Nurse Ratchet again. Don't bite your tongue, I tell myself. "I'd like to request a different nurse, if that's possible," I say, heart beating wildly.

"I'll tell my boss," the attendant says.

Moments later, the supervisor asks me why. I tell her about the previous week's experience and she assigns another nurse who's warm and attentive. But there are still problems: my lab work is delayed, even though the prescriptions for the labs *said* STAT. I learn that I need to say the tests are STAT, too. My new nurse can't start the infusion without the lab work. So we wait.

So much of living with cancer is waiting. Waiting for lab work. Waiting for appointments. Waiting for test results. Waiting to see what happens.

Tanya has prepared a picnic for us, so we don't have to eat hospital food. Soft rolls, tuna fish, celery, and organic Cheetos (because something salty during chemo tastes especially delicious.) The delay with the labs causes the treatment to last until early evening, so we have dinner, too: mozzarella cheese balls and cherry tomatoes with homemade vinaigrette, and juicy strawberries.

The nurses' station is right by my chair, and by the end of the day, we're all best friends. They tell me I'm spoiled. I nod. One of them asks, "What's your relationship?"

"We're married," I say.

They all brighten up.

"We've been together twenty-eight years," I add.

"But not legally married all that time, of course," Tanya says. "We got legally married last September."

They want to know all about the wedding and Cooper. We tell them that he just got a job offer, which he finally accepted today.

It's completely dark when we plod through our front door.

And now, after the second infusion, the side effects begin. Acne revisited. My face is completely covered with red pimples full of yellow pus. It doesn't resemble teenage acne. It's considerably worse. I float back in time to when I was fourteen. We lived in Hawaii then, and I had a crush on the lifeguard at the pool, a cute sailor who was probably nineteen. I remember swimming up through the water, slinking out of the pool in my bikini, and sauntering over to his stand, thinking my big brown eyes would look beautiful and he would notice. Instead, he asked me if I'd tried Lava soap for my pimples.

I'm not a vain person, but now my face is *so* bad that I don't even want to leave the house. If people are coming over, I warn them in advance, so they won't gasp when they come through the front door.

How long will this lovely side effect last?

Nobody knows.

I hibernate, even though it's spring and I yearn to be outside.

Cancer has chipped away at the edges of my life, shrunk it back to what's absolutely essential. Only the important aspects remain. In December 2007, before my diagnosis, I was busy all the time: work, more work, worry about work, social life, book group, girls' club, friends for coffee, friends for breakfast, conferences. Now, if there's more than one thing on my calendar in a day, I feel oppressed.

I feel boring from doing so little. I have nothing to say that's particularly interesting, unless I've been in the car and listened to NPR. It doesn't bother me a lot, just a little, but I used to think I was quite a conversationalist.

Each night after dark, Tanya and I sneak outside and walk around our neighborhood. The exercise energizes my body; the cool air on my hot, pimply face feels delicious. The night smells of jasmine, earthy and abundant.

April 8 arrives: Kim's last day at my office. We close the bank account. We terminate the business phone line and have the calls forwarded to my cell phone. We clear out the desk. We notify the State Bar that I'm going "inactive." We keep busy, busy, busy and make a plan to have lunch next week so we don't have to say goodbye today. Though I'll miss having Kim here on a regular basis, I'm completely relieved to have my business officially closed.

Coincidentally, it's also the first night of Passover, time for another Seder with Ann and John. In the past, there were sometimes more than twenty people, though in recent years, it's been more like twelve. This year, as promised, it's just Ann and John, Tanya and me.

At Stanford later in the week, Dr. Colevas says that if I were in the hospital, he'd have all his students check me out. "You're a perfect example of tumors dying from the inside out." Sounds good to me.

He looks at my red, inflamed face. "This is the worst Erbitux reaction I've seen," he says. "I'm going to take you off this drug." I'm both relieved and worried. What if it's the drug that's doing the good work?

And now, a few days after this treatment, still more side effects. My hair begins to fall out. It's globbed in the drain as I shampoo. Tanya's bare arm slips in and grabs it periodically, but the hair keeps coming out. I go to the salon and ask Angela to cut it very short. When she's done, I look adorable, but only if you can ignore my rash. The new look lasts only three days, when it becomes clear that there won't be enough hair left to look good. I go into the backyard, hang my head over the gravel, and Tanya shaves me until I'm bald. I've been here before. In fact, we're using the same electric shaver to shave my head that we used in 1986. Watching the hair fall to the ground is not as horrifying this time. But when I go upstairs and see myself in the mirror with all the pimples extending across my bald head, I burst into tears.

Several weeks later, my face is still red, inflamed, and bumpy and we're supposed to go to the Camp It Up twenty-year gala. All day, I worry about how to handle it. At 5 p.m. on the night of the party, I look in the mirror. The top half of my face is still red and pimply. The bottom half looks fine. I wash my face and peer at myself. I find some old makeup. Imagine that! The makeup covers *everything*. I look *almost* normal, though pasty pale. I put on my beautiful white silk blouse and my cool Japanese scarf over my bald head and feel great. The end of hibernation.

The event is fantastic. Lots of old-timers from the '90s. Good food. Rebecca Riots, a band that started at camp, plays a set. Then dancing, dancing, dancing. Tanya and I get to swing and move around the dance floor. Liberation.

But soon, I have to return to hibernation because my white blood count is dangerously low. "Don't even drive down here next Friday," Dr. Colevas says. "Your counts will be too low to get more chemo." He tells me I need to be very careful. My immune system is *extremely* compromised. I shouldn't be around anyone who is sick.

Since everyone I know is sick, I stay home. Marcie, my acupuncturist, makes a home visit so I don't have to come into her germy office for a treatment. I talk to my doctor Gabriella by phone. I skip my girls' club and check in with my friends by speakerphone.

But I go to Healing Man. I lie on his table on my side, and he does his ritual. His hands touch my back, my neck, my head. They are hot with energy. He guides me to connect to healing sources. I enter a semi-trance in which my body is totally rested and at peace, my mind focused on the white blood cells streaming up from my lower back into my body. When we're done, I feel radiant.

On my vacation day from chemo, I check my voicemail and find a message from my friend Mary. "Call me tonight if you can." The call came in last night. I call all her numbers, work, cell, girlfriend's, but she doesn't answer. I leave messages, but I already know that she's calling about a mutual friend and I know the news is not good, or she would have left a message.

Fortunately, Mary returns my call quickly. She reports that our friend has breast cancer.

I think about Mary, with two close friends grappling with cancer.

I think about our friend, who's in her sixties and still working hard as a lawyer.

I think about all she'll go through, but I feel certain she'll be okay.

As for myself, I imagine arising from a chair and walking forward into the version of myself in 2021. I merge with her. Light emanates from me.

SETTLING DOWN

I sit on the gray couch in the minuscule living room of our house on Albany Hill with Cooper on my lap. He's two months old. It's the end of April 1986 and I have one more month of maternity leave. Tanya is back at work today for the first time since Cooper was born. It feels strange to be home alone with our baby. I'm used to having Tanya's help.

The playpen we were given at his baby shower is folded up, standing in the corner. For some reason, I imagine Cooper standing up in it and almost gasp when I realize that once the playpen is opened, it will take up all the floor space in the living room. We'll have to step into the middle of the playpen and then back out again to get from the sofa to the rest of the house. I panic.

In truth, it required all the emotional energy I had to make the decision to have a baby and then to be pregnant. I didn't think much beyond that, except to find daycare for when I return to work.

And instead of focusing on all I don't know, or acknowledging the enormity of what we've embarked upon, or figuring out all I need to learn, I focus on what I think I can control, which is where we live, and I'm absolutely certain that we can't raise a family in our small one-bedroom house on Albany Hill. Our idea of making a tiny room in the basement for Cooper now seems ridiculous, with all those dangerously steep steps and the need to duck to avoid the header on the way down. What were we thinking?

I call Tanya at her law office. I tell her about the playpen. "We have to buy a new house," I announce. "We can't raise Cooper here. It's too small."

"Okay," she says, as if this is no big deal. "Start looking."

That night we decide on Berkeley. Albany has a reputation of being somewhat conservative. We decide that we want to be within ten blocks of the Monterey Market, our favorite produce store where we buy fresh lettuce, plump organic tomatoes, and creamy yogurt. For weeks, there's not a single house on the market.

Finally, the perfect home comes on the market, for sale by owner. Once we tour it, it occurs to us that the sellers might not want to sell to us. They've lived in the neighborhood for many years, have three kids, and are moving to the suburbs because they believe the schools are better there. We figure they'll want Ozzie and Harriet to replace them in their old home, not Harriet and Harriet.

We design a strategy: Tanya will look at the house a second time and take her law partner, Dan. She dresses in her best clothes—a long knit skirt, fancy boots, a silk blouse—and Dan wears a lawyer suit. I stay at home with Cooper in my gray sweats and flannel maternity shirt.

Tanya and Dan think the house is just right, in a great location with enough space to expand our family when Tanya is ready to get pregnant. It's in reasonable condition with a wonderful backyard.

Against our realtor's advice, we bid $20,000 over the asking price, and it's ours.

I grew up as a Navy brat. My family moved every year or two, and even after I graduated from high school and had some control over my life, I continued the habit of wandering. Three years is the longest I've ever lived in one place, in Norfolk, Virginia, when I was in first, second, and third grades. Counting dorm rooms and summer rentals, our new house will be my thirty-fourth residence in thirty-eight years. I'm excited. The first time I felt connected to a community as an adult, like I might stay a while, was when David and I built our yurt on our land in Ukiah. After coming out, though, I felt I couldn't go back. Buying this home in Berkeley feels like settling down again.

But just before escrow closes, when Cooper is only three months old, I'm diagnosed with lymphoma.

WISHFUL THINKING

It's late spring, a year and a half since my original tongue cancer diagnosis in January 2008 and five months since I was told I'm terminal. Dealing with my health has been a full-time job for seventeen months. The doorbell rings. Jane, who's been a friend for over twenty-five years, hugs me hello, talks briefly with Tanya, and leaves. Back at my desk, I'm attempting to create order out of chaos. Since I can't control my health, I want to exert control over something.

Home alone in the quiet house while Tanya does errands, I wander through the living room and spot on the couch Joan Didion's book *The Year of Magical Thinking*. One of my favorite books, it's a poignant memoir about Didion's experience of the death of her beloved husband and intellectual mate. I read it before I was diagnosed with cancer and was inspired to try writing creative nonfiction instead of fiction.

I can tell by the book jacket that what I'm looking at is not my copy. I wonder about that. Why's it here?

"Did Jane bring this book for me?" I ask Tanya when she comes home.

"No, she brought it for me."

The breath goes out of me, as if I've been punched. "I can't believe this. She must be planning for me to die! What's she *thinking*?" The last thing I would give Tanya to read, even if I *am* dying, would be Joan Didion's book. She's been busy reading *The Joy of Living* by

Yongey Mingyur Rinpoche, a Tibetan monk. She doesn't need a book about the grief of losing a spouse.

At least, not yet.

And then I remember how Jane responded the first time I had cancer. My intuition told me then that she was expecting me to die and that she had fantasies of moving right into my family to take my place. She'd always had a little crush on Tanya and later admitted she'd had such thoughts. It took several years after I recovered from lymphoma before Tanya and I completely re-established our relationship with her; she's endearing, generous, and loyal.

It dawns on me that not everyone shares my experience of my illness. I feel panicky at the thought that lots of folks think I'm dying and are simply indulging me in my fantasy of getting a miracle. Is everyone just humoring me while they wait for my imminent demise?

A few days later, Tanya and I are at Stanford at the PICC line department. After several months of weekly infusions of chemotherapy, my veins are destroyed. Last week, it took an hour and a half to get a vein started for my chemo! The nurses told me that I needed a PICC line, which is a skinny tube that will run inside a vein in my arm into my chest. Blood will be drawn and chemo will be administered through the line. No more needles poking into my bruised, scarred arms. I've reluctantly agreed to the PICC, but I'm nervous about getting it installed.

The nurse comes to get us, her lips smacking. "I'm eating a doughnut. I know I shouldn't, but I can't help myself. It's only a half." She's short, cute. Perky. Even though she's sixty, which she tells me when she sees from my chart that I'm also sixty.

She uses an ultrasound machine to find the vein and shows it to me on a monitor. The line goes in and we watch it snaking into my chest. First, it takes a wrong turn and detours into my neck. The nurse tells me to move my head into a different position, and the tube slithers into my chest. All the while, I feel nothing. Amazing!

The next day, I get dosed with multiple chemicals through my new PICC line. We leave Stanford in bright sun. "You wait," I say to Tanya. "It'll be foggy at our house." I'm completely grumpy. Driving to Stanford two days in a row has worn me out. It's three hours, at a minimum, on busy freeways with narrow lanes. In rush hour, it's even longer.

"It'll burn off," Tanya replies, ever optimistic.

I doze. Back in Berkeley, the sun is still shining.

"You wait," I say as I look up toward the hills. Sure enough, just two short blocks from our house, the fog is thick as mushroom soup and doesn't lift for the rest of the day. But I mostly sleep and read and ignore it as much as I can.

On a Sunday morning in late May 2009, we're at our little cabin on the Russian River. Despite all our efforts, it's still not sold. Desperate for financial relief, we decided to turn it into a vacation rental to help defray costs until the market is better. Tanya is madly getting it ready. Depleted, I'm just the cheerleader.

The fog has settled in. I sense it hanging over my head and struggle with my mind. I feel dragged down, as if I'm walking around in gray cotton.

Outside, the muddy river flows to the ocean. Trees are budding, but it's still dark, drippy, and wintery. I continue to be upset that Jane left Joan Didion's book for Tanya, and I decide to send her an email to tell her that I don't understand why she would give the book to Tanya right now. "I'm not preparing to die," I write. "Nor is Tanya preparing for me to die at this moment. We may come to that, but that's not what's happening now. It feels like you might be in a different place with this."

Jane responds that she doesn't understand what my prognosis is, because the last thing she heard was that I had six to nine months to live. "I know you are remaining positive and not wanting to talk about the cancer, but I feel some frustration about not knowing what is going on."

It seems to me that she doesn't understand the complexity of trying to live each day with the possibility of an early death lingering in the air. All the emails I've sent to my cancer list, which she's on, haven't penetrated.

Before I can respond, she sends a second email: "I realize that I made a serious error in judgment. I've been thinking it over a lot and I am not happy about it. I hope you will forgive me. . ."

Ah, the power of the sincere apology. "I understand that supporting me in my ambiguous state is not easy," I write back. "A different Western medicine prognosis would make it much simpler for all of us. But we're dealing with what we're dealing with, and I remain full of hope and vigor at the moment."

Connecting with important longtime friends is part of my healing. Back home from our river cabin, my friend Susan and I spread out in the living room reminiscing and catching up on each other's life. Susan and I met when we both worked in the family planning clinic in Ukiah in the early 1970s. She was a women's health-care specialist; I was a clinic assistant. We did health and birth control education for women. "You know, I was as happy at that job as I've ever been," I say.

"We were such a good team, weren't we?" she says.

"With the world's worst boss." Our boss gave us no room to be creative or to develop new programs. We were young and full of ideas. All she said was no. "Think what it could have been with a good boss."

We talk about the two years we lived together at 22nd and Irving in San Francisco later in the '70s when I was still in law school. It was such a lovely life. I drove commute buses; by then a lapsed physician's assistant, she drove tour buses. We crossed paths every day over tea or dinner.

How magical the '70s were, I think, noticing for the first time that most of my closest friends come from that time.

It's June, and time for another update to my cancer list. I can't possibly see everyone and maintain my health. My time is devoured by doctor's appointments with Gabriella, body work with Jill, acupuncture with Marcie, a daily hour-long homeopathy ritual, walking, resting, Healing Man, Stanford, travel to and from appointments, organizing and taking multitudes of supplements, meditation. Writing the email updates keeps people in the loop and keeps me from having to tell everyone the news.

"I read daily," I write. "Lots of *New Yorkers*. Some wonderful books. I write." I tell them that the chemo is ongoing, with relatively minor side effects except fatigue and the rash, which has been slow to heal. The good news is that the tumors "have shrunk or disappeared altogether."

Then I write the most important part, the part that's designed to keep people from asking me questions about the medical process. "People seem to have lots of questions," I write. "I have no answers. I continue to avoid spending time talking about my disease. This has actually been quite liberating since previously, people wanted more and more medical information, which increased everyone's anxiety. My oncologist approaches this week by week, and doesn't do a lot of projecting forward about what's next, because that depends upon what's happening next week, and the week after that, which we can't know. So, it's another lesson in living in the moment, not controlling everything, and enjoying life—being in joy—as much as possible."

Later in the week, Jane, who gave Tanya the Didion book, telephones. Despite having read my email, she's filled with questions: Is your hair still gone? Yes. Do you still have your rash? 85% gone. When you touch your face, can you feel it? No, but there are holes. Like pock marks? I guess so. I'm now ready to scream. It seems like she's more worried about how I look than how I feel. Do I need this? Where's the line between forgiveness and taking care of myself? Where's the line between "doing no harm" to others and doing no harm to myself?

Are they going to give you the chemical that causes the rash again? I don't know. We go moment by moment. We decide what to do each week. Now I'm grinding my teeth.

"It must be hard living in the moment," she finally says. "I like to plan."

I bite my tongue. I'd like to say that it's easier to live in the moment when the sun is shining, which it hasn't done in weeks. And when the people around me are able to accept ambiguity and their own mortality. But this is Jane being Jane, saying just what's in her mind without filtering it. I know she means well.

I'm skimming through the *Chronicle* in early June when I come across this headline: "Susan Jordan—lawyer took on SLA, activist cases." My chest constricts. My eyes water. Susan died in a plane crash at age sixty-seven, I learn. "She . . . gained fame for a landmark case of rape victim Inez Garcia, who was convicted of killing one of her attackers. In a 1977 retrial, Ms. Jordan won Garcia's acquittal on grounds that she acted in self-defense."

Susan was the professor teaching Criminal Procedure when I visited New College in 1977 and one of the main reasons I chose to go there for law school. That was over thirty years ago. I graduated from law school, got divorced, and *left* Ukiah just as Susan moved her practice *to* Ukiah, where she continued to practice criminal law until her death.

I'm alive, dancing with cancer. She's died in a plane crash.

Who lives and who dies is random.

Another day at Stanford. I go every week. It's an unusual regimen that Dr. Colevas decided upon for me. Usually, chemo is every three or four weeks but I'm getting smaller doses on a weekly basis instead.

Last week, Dr. Colevas complained about a David Foster Wallace book he was trying to read. "It's so hard to get through," he'd said.

"I have trouble reading Wallace, too. But life is too short to waste time reading a book you don't love," I said. "You ought to know this in your line of work!"

He wrote down the name of a book I suggested, *Fugitive Pieces,* and put it in his wallet. "You don't understand," he said. "I never give up on a book. What will happen is that someone will want the book and the library will make me return it because I've renewed it so many times and still not finished it."

"Maybe I'll do that to let you off the hook."

Today, he comes in the examining room without the usual hello. "Did you go to the Palo Alto library and request the David Foster Wallace book?"

I laugh out loud. "Absolutely not."

"I don't believe you," he laughs. "Someone actually requested it and I had to return it. But that book you recommended isn't in."

I love it that my doc goes to the library.

I haven't had chemotherapy for two weeks, and fully expect to get it today, but my white blood count is still too low. Dr. Colevas orders shots to stimulate white blood cell production. The problem: the shots are so expensive that the insurance company has to pre-approve them. This will take time. I worry about the lapse in getting treatment. Does this let the cancer cells proliferate?

Tanya and I go to the pharmacy and wait. And wait. And wait. After two hours, I go to the counter to ask whether they have approval. One of the pharmacists suggests that I call Blue Cross myself. I feel so weak and so overwhelmed, I'm close to tears. I go outside to get reception on my cell phone and call Blue Cross.

"Your doctor needs to call and ask that this be expedited," the man on the line says.

"How long will it take then?" I ask.

"Maybe tomorrow."

"This is crazy," I say. "I know it's not your fault, but I'm at Stanford. I have cancer. I live an hour and a half away. I need to be instructed about how to inject this drug. I can't drive all the way back down here tomorrow."

He gives me a bureaucratic response.

And I blow up. "I repeat: I *know* this isn't your fault, but this is just *BULLSHIT*. It's no way to treat a person who's sick and in the middle of chemotherapy."

I'm in a rage. I don't do this often. I know it doesn't make the medical establishment work better. I know it's not good for my immune system. I know it doesn't even make *me* feel better. But I am completely out of reserves and unable to contain myself. I go back to the clinic and ask to see Dr. Colevas's assistant, who calms me down and says it will probably be approved this afternoon.

After another hour, I have the drug and I'm perfecting my shot technique.

Moments later, we get respite. Tanya and I bask in the afternoon sun at Tootsie's, a café near the hospital. Hundreds of bees swarm in the lavender surrounding the patio. The sun is penetrating, but the air is cool. And for *just* a moment, I feel like a normal person.

We wend our way home in Friday afternoon traffic, and at 7:00 p.m. the phone rings. "Ms. Reaves, this is Dr. Colevas."

"You can definitely call me Martina at this point," I say for probably the fiftieth time. "You're working late. What's up?"

"I've been thinking about your counts," he says. "You're robust. It doesn't make sense that it's taking so long for your counts to go back up. There are the explanations we talked about, that you've had a lot of chemotherapy and you may be fighting a cold, but I just have this niggling feeling. I need to know more about the supplements you're taking."

He's always joking with me about my supplement list and the homeopathy I take. I get out my list and read it to him. It's long and, frankly, difficult to manage, not to mention expensive.

"How would you feel if I asked you to stop taking three things: the mushrooms and the two prescriptions of Chinese herbs?"

I'm moved by how respectful he is; that he doesn't *order* me to stop.

"No problem," I say.

A week later, I pack my bags to be gone all day at Stanford. I take several issues of *The New Yorker, The Winter Vault,* my current book, *The Week,* our favorite board game (Sequence), bottles of alkaline water that I've started drinking, my shawl, my own fuzzy brown blanket that Tanya gave me for Christmas. After all these months, I *finally* figured I should bring my own blanket instead of huddling under those thin white hospital blankets that pill all over my black pants.

I'm oddly relaxed as we leave the house to drive down, even though I know that today is the day for the results of another PET scan they did a few days ago.

How many bad test results have I gotten since all this started in January 2008? Too many to count, I think.

"I want to plant a vegetable garden in the backyard," I say to Tanya as we drive toward the freeway. I've been talking to her about this for several weeks. About how we should do this when we get our river cabin set up as a vacation rental, which seems to be taking forever. "Maybe Cooper could help us on Sunday."

"I was hoping to get Cooper to go to the cabin with us again this weekend to do some more work," Tanya says.

I'm sick of the cabin, the to-do lists, the time and energy it has taken. "I can't think of anything I want to do less," I say.

I'm met with silence.

"No comment?" I ask. Before she can respond, I get mad. "Look, you're always telling me to figure out what I want, and here I've figured it out, and when I put it out, you don't respond." I'm on a roll. I say more.

Finally, Tanya says, "I can't do this now. I can't drive to Stanford and have a fight."

"Okay, I understand that. I'll stop talking, then."

I sit quietly, surprised by the intensity of my anger. I breathe deeply and wonder whether this is displaced anxiety about getting my test results.

We listen to NPR. When we hit San Leandro, Tanya asks, "What do you want to plant?"

"I can't talk about this now," I say. I'm still angry.

What a time to have a fight, I think. This is an unusual event. Tanya and I haven't fought very often while I've been sick.

I think about how she is a person who *always* knows what she wants, that I'm a person who is *always* ambivalent and unsure. Waiting around for me to figure out what I want drives her crazy. On a Saturday morning, she's up and ready to go. I wake up slowly, want to make up the bed, tidy the house, eat, drink a cup of tea, putter.

Then, maybe, I can begin to think about what might be fun. We've struggled with this difference for twenty-eight years, and we mostly work it out. But not today.

By the time we get to Stanford, I've calmed myself down with the thought of not wanting high blood pressure when they take my readings. Breathe in. Breathe out. Breathe in. First to the infusion room for a blood draw and a dressing change for my PICC line. Then to Clinic A to see Dr. Colevas.

Jamie, his assistant, comes into the examining room. I remind her that I've gotten a CT scan and a PET CT scan. "I'll check them now," she says.

She pulls the results up on the screen. I realize that I could simply get up and read over her shoulder and find out what the results are, but I stay in my seat. She turns to us. "I like to give results when they're good," she says, smiling. "Nothing shows up on the PET CT. Nothing. Of course, Dr. Colevas will want to take a look at this and tell you more. He'll be in soon."

I can hardly believe it. I sneak a peek at Tanya. She's ecstatic.

Jamie leaves Tanya and me alone, and we look at each other with feelings that are too complicated to name.

I have imagined this, the moment when I'm told that no cancer shows up on the scan. I know that this doesn't mean I'm cured, at least so far as the medical establishment is concerned. They think that there are millions of little cells waiting to grow, that they're just too small to show up on the scan. But I think that maybe all this work I've been doing is having an effect.

Dr. Colevas confirms what Jamie has said. "The scans show no tumor. That area that was swelling behind your ear is smaller and there's no sign of tumor there, either. I want to give you a few more treatments, just to be sure. A few meaning two to four. And another round of the injections to keep your white blood count up. Your counts today are fine."

At the infusion room, Nurse Jackie, a Filipina whose real name, she says, is Rosemarie, is my nurse for the day. She uses Jackie because there's another Rosemarie. Instead of picking a chair in the big room with lots of other chemo patients, I pick a private room. The upside to this is the privacy. The downside is that there are no windows.

Jackie and I chat as she gets things ready. Next week, she and her husband are going to the Philippines for a two-week vacation with their two children, ages four and eight. The last time they visited, the eight-year-old was a baby. She wants to know if I have a child and is happy to hear that I do.

I snuggle in under my fuzzy brown blanket. She brings lots of pills. Some patients are very interested in everything they are taking and study each item carefully. I look, to satisfy the nurse, but the truth is I'm not really that interested in the details. After the pills, the bags arrive to be dripped into my veins: 50 milligrams of Benadryl, to keep me from having an allergic reaction.

I go into a stupor. Sleep. Total relaxation. I'm gone for two or three hours while Tanya goes on escapades. She brings me a new style of hat from the gift store. She walks to Andronico's at the Stanford Shopping Center and brings lunch. She makes phone calls to deliver the good news to my mother, her mother, our friends. When I wake up, we play gin rummy.

I'm floating, from the wonderful news, from the drugs, from getting to rest after a busy week. Late in the afternoon, the last drip goes in, and we drive home.

The next morning, I wake up with two thoughts: "I don't have cancer," and "The body wants to heal," which is what Marcie, my acupuncturist, always says. Butterflies flutter in my stomach.

I sit on the back deck in my shirtsleeves and feel like I'm on vacation. My thoughts drift. The sun burns. What do I do with myself? I know that Dr. Colevas thinks I still have lots of little cancer seeds just waiting to sprout, but I'm putting my sprouting energy into the garden we just planted: all kinds of lettuces and cherry tomatoes. Later, we'll plant spinach, chard, and arugula.

I'm choosing to think that the cancer is gone. Wishful thinking? Thoughtful wishing? We'll have to wait to see.

OUR SOUTHERN CONNECTIONS

Cooper is nine months old, and since his birth in February, my life has been turned upside down: I've become a mother, survived intense chemotherapy for lymphoma and a hospitalization for pneumonia, resigned my law partnership, and moved into our new house. I've barely recuperated as we board the flight to Texas to visit Tanya's family. My hair is soft, baby fine, barely two inches long, and I have about a quarter inch of stamina.

We've made a family, and Tanya wants to show it off to her family of origin, despite her father's comment about Cooper being a bastard and knowing how conservative many of them are.

I've already watched Tanya break out in mounds of fever blisters every time she goes to Texas for a visit, so I'm not enthusiastic. For one thing, I'll be meeting the famous Aunt Celestine.

I know *all* about Celestine because The Celestine Stories filled many hours of our time when Tanya and I were first getting to know each other. Celestine is Tanya's aunt, her father Nelson's sister. When Tanya's parents got married in 1947, Tanya's sister Jimmie Lee was two. Nelson adopted her, but Aunt Celestine didn't consider Jimmie Lee real "family" because she wasn't related to Nelson by blood. At the time, Aunt Celestine was still single and desperately wanted to have a child in her life, so she encouraged Tanya's parents to have their own baby and promised to help in every way, including financially.

Laura and Nelson agreed, and Tanya is the result.

Fierce, judgmental, controlling, and generous, Aunt Celestine is the epitome of the shriveled Southern spinster. She was also an assistant to a federal judge, an independent woman, and a role model. And she dotes on Tanya.

After Tanya became a lawyer, Celestine began pestering her about whether she had "a young man." Finally, sometime in 1979, Tanya wrote her a long letter that said she was going to be a professional, unmarried woman *just* like Celestine, although she wasn't quite ready to come out. As if in response, months later, just before she turned sixty, Celestine married Sledge Clinkscales, a friend she'd known since childhood. It was her first marriage.

Just after the marriage, Tanya's therapist said that she wanted to meet with Celestine and Tanya together. By then, Tanya had come out to her family. As Celestine told Tanya upon her arrival in California, "You've never asked me to do anything, so when you asked me to come to therapy with you, of course I said, 'Yes.'"

As Tanya tells the story, the session with the therapist lasted a short five minutes. The therapist asked Celestine if she wanted to discuss Tanya's homosexuality. Celestine reared back and snorted, "Absolutely not!" And that ended the session.

I'm definitely not looking forward to meeting Aunt Celestine.

I'm also apprehensive about meeting Tanya's father and his wife Jo for the first time.

The only person I'm looking forward to seeing is Tanya's sister Jimmie Lee, who flew to California to help us with Cooper for a few weeks after I was diagnosed. But all in all, I'm making this trip with great reluctance.

Our flight is a disaster. Cooper is feverish with horrible diarrhea. Wouldn't you know, I'm exhausted by the time we arrive.

Tanya's father picks us up at the airport and drives us to his house in Beaumont, which is an hour and a half outside Houston. Beaumont is about as ugly as anyplace I've ever been in the world and definitely *not* the "beautiful mountain" its name would suggest. It's flat, filled with strip malls, neon signs (one of which is a big red arrow flashing "JESUS HERE"), ranch houses, churches (of all denominations you've heard of, like Baptist, Lutheran, Methodist, and Catholic, and many you've never heard of, like Word of Faith and Alpha and Omega), big cars, and unbelievably horrible food (limp, over-cooked vegetables, lots of meat dripping in BBQ sauce, and white Styrofoam bread). But it's where Tanya's family moved when she was seven, and, coincidentally, where my parents spent the first night of their honeymoon after they married in Houston in 1939.

Tanya has choreographed our entire trip. Her parents divorced when she was in college, so we have to divide our time between their two homes. When we first arrive, we stay with Nelson and his second wife, Jo. Her father married Jo just as Tanya finished law school, when she was twenty-three.

The morning after our arrival, I sit at the kitchen table with Cooper nestled in my arms. Tanya is next to me. Nelson is at the head of the table and Jo serves us all as we wait for Aunt Celestine to appear.

With all the Celestine stories tucked away, I'm nervous to meet her. She walks into the dining room, impeccably dressed, hair perfectly coiffed and lacquered, lipstick and rouge in place. She looks at me, completely ignores Cooper, whom she's not met yet, scowls, sits down, and sniffs, "Well, if I'd known how Tanya would turn out, I *never* would have helped her go to law school."

I take a deep breath. "I think she turned out pretty great," I say, as perkily as I can. Celestine glares.

"How was your flight?" she asks. And after we handle *that* question, the conversation turns to the weather when we left California. As I come to learn, the weather is a *big* topic in Texas.

In fact, it's all we talk about until Tanya and I pack up and move to Tanya's mother's house. Tanya's mother Laura is also remarried, to a man named Earl. There is more polite conversation about the weather, of course, and the plane trip and Cooper. Nobody mentions my health, my work, or the changes in my life. When I inquire of Tanya why nobody is talking to me, Tanya laughs, "That would be rude."

On Thanksgiving, we converge on Tanya's sister Jimmie Lee's house. The smell of butter, yeasty biscuits, and onions wafts out the front door as we arrive. Jimmie Lee's husband, Big Joe, glances at us from his lounge chair in the living room, but he doesn't say hello or greet us in any way. He's called Big Joe to distinguish him from his son Little Joe, aka Joe Joe. All four of Jimmie Lee's children line up in a row and greet us warmly—Shelly and Robin (wearing tight sweaters and blue jeans topped with big Farrah Fawcett hair, pancake makeup, and lots of eye shadow and mascara) and Chip and Joe Joe (with hair combed and clean T-shirts).

Jimmie Lee has obviously been working for days to prepare the elaborate spread: The table shimmers with family serving dishes, silverware, and heavy cranberry-colored crystal plates and glasses. When it's time for the meal, Big Joe sits ceremoniously at the head of the table, but never says a word as the rest of us ooh and aah over the food. In fact, I never hear his voice the entire afternoon.

I paste a smile across my face and use my best manners, the ones my grammy taught me that I hardly ever have to use anymore. Our celebrations in California are never this formal. It's just not our style.

That night, I have a vivid nightmare: I'm locked up in a room with white padded walls and my captors aren't going to let me out, no matter what I do or say. The dream is so intense, I'm anxious long after I wake up. I'm clammy; my stomach flutters; I'm nauseous. Utterly exhausted from traveling, from still waking up at night with Cooper, from the aftermath of chemo and cancer, I positively dread the prospect of three more days in Beaumont.

"I've made a decision," I say to Tanya when she wakes up. "I'm going to be sick with the flu now. You're going to go to the drugstore to buy me some mysteries and I'm going to stay in this bedroom until we leave."

Which is exactly what I do.

NOW WHAT?

It's a few months after Kim has stopped working for me, toward summer, and we're celebrating her birthday. She arrives promptly at 6 p.m., dressed in her legal secretary clothes: sandals, red toenails, makeup, black slacks and a jacket. Her skin glows, smooth and perfect. Her long hair is pulled back and held in place with a barrette. It's incomprehensible that someone can look this good after the day she's had.

Recently separated from her husband, Mark, she's moved out of their home and gotten a new full-time job at a law firm in Oakland after years of working part-time for Tanya and me. Yesterday, she moved into a rental house and slept there alone last night. This morning, she picked up three of her kids at Mark's house, took them to two schools in different locations, drove to BART, and caught a train to arrive at work in Oakland by nine.

Now, nine hours later, she looks elegant, but she clunks into the house in her high-heeled sandals, hugs us both, and collapses inelegantly onto the couch.

"What do you want to drink?" Tanya asks.

"White wine."

"What do you want, Martina?"

"I'm thinking." I'm into my familiar state of ambivalence. Even though the doctor says I can drink now, I'm not in the mood. "I'll just have water," I say.

Kim fills us in. "I need to get things from the house, but Mark says I've 'abandoned' it, and that everything is his. I don't know who he's talking to, but it's bad advice. I wrote him a long letter today, telling him the stuff we bought while we were together is owned fifty-fifty. He's acting like someone I don't know. I never would have predicted all the shit he's doing."

"You know that this is the time when people lose control," I say. "It's not worth having a big fight over the stuff. Please be careful." Kim is five-foot-two; her husband is a big, burly Irish guy who likes to drink.

"We have lots of stuff we don't need," Tanya says to Kim as she heads up to the attic. She returns bearing gifts. Old stainless-steel kitchen utensils we were saving for Cooper. Wine glasses we don't need. Sheets. Bedspreads.

Tanya signals to me to come into the kitchen. "Is it okay to give her these?" She's holding a set of delicate translucent porcelain bowls and a matching cream pitcher with hand-painted strawberries on them. I laugh and nod yes.

"Here's our present to you and your girls," Tanya says. "I got them when I first graduated from law school in 1977."

"And I couldn't believe she had them when we first met," I laughed. "They were *way* too femme for me. Like tea party stuff my grammy had."

"My girls will *love* them," Kim says. She's grateful to have presents to take home to her mostly empty house.

As Kim requested, we go to Venezia for dinner. The restaurant has walls painted with scenes from Venice. Clothes hang from laundry lines crisscrossing the ceiling. Fountains splash water. I love the feeling of being transported somewhere else. I spy a purple bra that wasn't hanging last time I ate here and realize that the clothes on the lines have been changed for the summer season. Such attention to detail!

More Mark talk.

"I swore I wasn't going to burden the two of you with all my divorce talk," Kim says.

"What are friends for? It's what's happening. What else would we talk about?" Honestly, who better to talk to than me, a family lawyer and a mediator? During my career, I must have talked to hundreds of people in Kim's situation. It feels familiar.

"Well, I have a great story for you," Kim says. "And it's not about the divorce. I was staying at my friend's house in Benicia with the kids last week before my rental was ready. We were all lounging in the bedroom and Chelsea came over and handed me my cell phone with a text message on it." Chelsea is Kim's sixteen-year-old daughter.

"I looked at the phone," Kim continues, "and the message said, 'I like girls.' I was totally confused and couldn't figure out where it had come from, and then I realized that it was a text from Chelsea. She was trying to tell me something important. I looked at her and said, 'I kinda thought so.'"

Tanya and I are howling. Coming out, 2009-style. We'd always thought Chelsea was in the "family," so we're not surprised.

"Wait," Kim says. She's doubled over from laughing. "It goes on. I was still thinking about Chelsea when another text came in. Sydney handed me the phone." Sydney is Kim's thirteen-year-old daughter. "'What now?' I said. The text was from Sydney, and said, 'Don't worry, Mom, I'm straight.'"

When we stop laughing, the conversation gets more serious. "Chelsea's only in tenth grade. You know how it is where I live. I'm really worried she'll get harassed," Kim says. Kim only lives twenty minutes from Berkeley, but it's considerably more conservative there.

"Well, who has she told about this?" I ask.

"Only me and Sydney."

"Maybe that's all she's going to do for now," I say. "Let her take her time."

We each order salad and pasta with prawns, and now I cut loose. I haven't touched alcohol in a year and half, except at our wedding in September 2008, when I had a sip of champagne that tasted horrible. Slowly, ever so slowly, my taste buds have come back to life. I order my first drink, a gin and tonic, and it tastes delicious—cold, smooth, tart. It sparkles in the glass, liquid light.

"So, now I have a story for you. I've got to tell you about what happened with my husband after I told him I wanted a divorce," I say.

"Go for it," Kim says.

"Before he was with me, he was an Episcopal priest and lived in Greenwich, Connecticut, outside New York, commuting into Manhattan on the train like Don Draper. While we were married, he was a hippie, a streetcar driver, and worked for nonprofits that helped kids. Within a week after I told him I wanted a divorce, he cut me off medical insurance, despite some pre-existing medical issues and the fact that I didn't have a job. In all the years I've been a lawyer, I've only seen one other man do this to his wife."

"So what did you do?"

"I borrowed money from my parents and studied for the bar exam. Within two weeks, he was sleeping with the church secretary. She'd moved to Ukiah from Southern California with her husband and three kids because, as she told David, 'God told her there was a priest in Ukiah who needed her.' When she arrived in town, she went from church to church to figure out which priest God had in mind for her. She found David and began working as his secretary in the year prior to our separation. In a matter of months, she and David got into speaking in tongues and all the born-again stuff."

Kim listens intently.

"The last thing I heard about him was from a newspaper clipping from the *San Diego Union* that my mother sent me more than ten years ago," I say. "It described three Episcopal priests who were leaving the Episcopal Church and renouncing their vows to protest the ordination of women and homosexuals."

"During our marriage," I continue, "David acted like a left-wing hippie and a feminist, but within months of our separation, he was another person altogether. I think it's weird how people seem to change after a break-up and how they act in ways that seem out of character. I *never* would have thought that David would change in the ways he did."

I tell Kim what Ann says about this topic, that it's the effect of the chemistry of attraction. When two people are together, they bring out parts of each other. When they split up, other parts emerge that weren't part of that chemistry.

"But," I tell Kim, "what I think is that some people are chameleons and become like the people they spend time with. Their inner cores are not developed. You brought out the best parts of Mark. Now he's with people who encourage his less pleasant traits."

A few days later, at another Healing Man appointment, I receive a new prescription: "Smile. Make your lips reach your ears. Even if you don't feel it. Rehearse it. When you smile, your toes feel it. They start wagging their tails, like a cat."

Tanya, sitting in a chair next to me, blue eyes twinkling, laughs out loud.

On July 10, 2009, I tell Dr. Colevas, "This is my last chemotherapy treatment, unless, of course, you say something that changes my mind today."

In fact, it was all I could do to drag myself to this appointment. I'm completely depleted; almost sixty pounds lighter than when I was diagnosed. When I'm naked, my flesh hangs off bones and I look ancient, like my mother who's almost ninety, like a person who's starving to death.

"Why have chemo today, then?" he asks.

"Because I'm superstitious. Four weeks ago, you said you wanted to do two to four more treatments. This will be number four. I'm ready to do it."

"Would you be willing to say that this is the last one *for now?* So that you might entertain more in the future?" he asks.

"Yes, but I'm still calling it my last treatment." I smile at him. My toes are wagging their tails. I understand that he wants to prepare me for when it comes back again.

"I have a present for you," I say as I hand him *Fugitive Pieces.*

He looks at it, and starts to hand it back, saying, "You have to write in it."

"I already have." It says: "Thank you for your compassionate and respectful treatment. Don't spend time reading books you don't love, even this one!"

He reads it and smiles. "I'm getting on a red-eye tonight, and probably won't read it then. But maybe on the way back."

"No rush," I say.

"So, follow up. Do you want a short leash or a long one?" he asks.

We settle on a short leash, a return visit in mid-August. He writes the chemotherapy prescription for today and adds: "Patient to take bubble bath when she goes home." He knows that my body aches for one because I've been unable to take a bath since I got my PICC line months ago.

I plod to the elevator that will take me upstairs to the infusion room because climbing the stairs just one flight is more energy than I can muster. I want to be done with chemo. I crave it. I want the PICC line out of my arm.

Sounds of chemotherapy: The white noise of the air system, always a constant. The rhythmic scrunch, scrunch, scrunch of the machine pumping chemicals into the line. The squeaks of rubber-soled shoes on the linoleum tiles in the hallway. The beeps of machines when they run out of chemo. The higher beeps of the nurses' call button. The whoosh of sliding glass doors opening and closing. The clunks of the metal door to the infusion room. The snoring of the man across the hall. The swishes of people walking down the hall. Every once in a while, if it's real quiet, the clicks of the second hand on the clock on the wall as it passes the minute hand. The mumbles of people talking in the infusion room. It's like a concert hall, lots of sound, but I can't discern a word. One little fart from me.

2:52 p.m. Body sensations: Slightly queasy stomach. Tingling fingers. Stiff, clunky feet. Dry nose. Sore back from lying in this bed for almost six hours. Antsy energy. I want out of here!

3:15 p.m.: We walk out of Stanford Cancer Clinic. Next appointment, August 14. I'm elated . . . and fragile.

A few days later, I go to Jill, my body worker, whom I've seen weekly during this entire ordeal. In the November surgery on my neck, a nerve and many muscles had to be cut out, and now my shoulder sags. Jill has worked with me diligently to keep my body in line and my muscles unknotted. I have two hours on the table.

Anxious thoughts rise up and invade my mind. Every little knot Jill works on in my neck makes me wonder if it's a cancer lymph node. My brain hooks onto worry just like that, in a second, unbidden.

I breathe deeply. I imagine the ocean, the tide pools, smells of seaweed and salt water. My body begins to relax. Jill digs deeper. She goes to places her fingers haven't gone in over a year.

More worry bubbles. What do I do now? More fistfuls of supplements? Sounds wrong. Too many pills. The strong Chinese herbs? They overwhelm my gut. There you go, thinking too hard. Stop. Breathe again. Listen to the music. I imagine that spring day running naked on the beach with my friend Tom, before he had AIDS, before I had cancer, when we were both still young and carefree. Then, I'm in a half-trance, until Jill touches me gently and tells me to move onto my side. When she's finally done, I have no pain anywhere in my body. At least for the moment.

Now what?

I don't have an answer, but I trust that one will come.

OUTSIDE THE BOX

From the moment of his birth, Cooper lives outside the box. A wild child, he's energetic, enthusiastic, kinetic, intense. He wants to *move*. No sitting down and being mellow. No babe in arms. No Madonna scenes with this boy. Get up, go outside, dance.

When he's six months old, we enroll him in a well-respected daycare program and he gets kicked out almost immediately. "We can't meet his needs," the director says. She's got six babies and two teachers in a room that's twenty-by-twenty feet. Cooper would need the entire room to himself, he's so active. She wants babies who sit in one place for fifteen minutes at a time. That's not our boy. And she wants kids who don't get ear infections. She wonders if Cooper's ear infections are related to my cancer. Her logic: pressure at home and pressure on the ear! So we move him into daycare with Jim who piles five kids into car seats in his old burgundy Buick and goes places: the beach, the park, mall-running when it rains. Nothing yuppie about this daycare. Half the time when we pick him up, Cooper tells us to go away, he's not ready to go home.

He climbs the six-foot fence in the backyard before he can walk, before he's one. He pulls out drawers in the kitchen to make stairs to climb up to the counter. He's always on the move.

Meanwhile, we struggle with systems that don't actually recognize our family. We revise every single form we have to fill out: At the doctor's office, we cross off "Father" and write in "Mother." At preschool, we explain that Tanya is to be treated as a parent. We have legal forms drafted so that Tanya can be Cooper's guardian if something happens to me. So far as the law is concerned, Tanya is considered a "legal stranger." No matter that he calls her Mom and that she *is* his mom.

This goes on until Cooper is four, in 1990. At this point, we think the time might be right to change things. A judge who's friendly to same-sex couples sits on the bench that handles adoptions in our county. We hire a lawyer and head to court.

The three of us sit in his courtroom in Alameda County. Tanya's mother sits behind us with several friends and Cooper's godfather from Australia. We're all nervous, except Cooper. He bounces from lap to lap, his usual exuberant self.

We're hoping that Judge Kawaichi will allow Tanya to legally adopt Cooper without requiring me to give up my parental rights. We're a test case in Alameda County to see if the law can be stretched to make both Tanya and me legal parents. We hear that another lesbian couple across the bay in San Francisco is making the same request in a San Francisco courtroom.

Our lawyer, Ginny Palmer, has written legal briefs giving the court all the reasons to do the right thing. She thinks the judge will do it, but you just never know. Through the grapevine, we learn that the social worker who has investigated our family is a Mormon. She interviewed us, Cooper, our friends, his teachers. We wonder if her religion will prejudice her against us, and are relieved when we see that she's written a very favorable report. However, the last paragraph recommends that the adoption not be granted because it is "the policy of the California Department of Social Services to recommend against same-sex parents." It's upsetting to think about all the fathers who are legal parents simply because their sperm created the child, even if they're not interested in their child at all. Nobody checks them out before letting them be a parent. The injustice rankles me.

The judge emerges from his chambers. We all rise. He sits and then we sit.

Our case is called. Tanya, Cooper, and I walk forward. I find myself shivering with anticipation. Ginny says, "Your Honor, as you'll see from the statements we have submitted, this is a true family in every sense. All these witnesses are here in court today to testify, if you like, to the quality of the parenting and the love in this household. We are asking you to declare Tanya Starnes the legal parent of Cooper Reaves, while permitting Martina Reaves to continue as his other legal parent. This child deserves the legal protection that having two parents will give him."

Judge Kawaichi responds by talking directly to Cooper, telling him how lucky he is to have two people who love him. *He's going to do it,* I think, and minutes later, he confirms Tanya as a parent.

I hadn't expected this to be an emotional experience. I had thought of it as simple paperwork. But when the judge says that we're both parents, tears stream down my face and I start shaking with emotion. I look around me. Almost everyone in the courtroom is crying, including the court clerks. We're a real family! Recognized by the state!

This is as close as I'm ever going to get, I think, (incorrectly, it will later turn out) to having my relationship with Tanya legally recognized.

Even after Cooper's adoption, we discover that we still need to educate people about our family. When it's time for kindergarten in 1991, we figure we might be the first two-mom family at Jefferson School. And as we all know, kindergarten involves talking about your family and your neighborhood. How will Cooper, who isn't a verbal giant, explain his family to his classmates?

"What do we do?" we ask a teacher friend.

"Easy," she says. "You write a letter and tell his teacher how to act, just like we tell the kids how to act. She'll do what you say."

And that's what we do. We write that Cooper has two mothers, that he calls each of us Mom, that he has a father he will meet when he's eighteen, and on and on and on, anticipating all the questions, and yes, we say, he lets us know which mother he's talking to or which mother he needs.

We take him to kindergarten the first day and cry all the way home.

The thing about being the first lesbian family in your neighborhood or school is that any time your child acts out, you fear that everyone will think it's because he's from a lesbian family. That it's because he doesn't have a father to "set him straight." That somehow you're doing something wrong. You feel eyes on you, wondering how your child will turn out. No matter how wonderful things are, lurking in the psychological landscape is a tiny sense that you don't truly belong.

Sometime during the first week of kindergarten, the phone rings. "This is Mrs. Altman's secretary. Is this Cooper's mom?"

Uh-oh, I think. Mrs. Altman is the principal. "Yes, this is Martina," I say.

"Don't worry, Cooper is okay, but Mrs. Altman needs to talk to you. Can you come to school?"

Tanya and I rush down together. Cooper sits contritely on an old wooden bench outside Mrs. Altman's office, his short legs swinging in the air above the floor. She calls all three of us inside. It seems that he has bitten another boy in his class and left teeth marks! We're horrified and assure her that he's never bitten anyone before, which is true. She looks at Cooper over the top of her bifocals and sternly tells him that he'd better not do it again. Quiet for once in his life, he mumbles that he won't.

We walk out of the principal's office with Cooper and his kindergarten teacher, who pulls us aside. "I'm not supposed to say this," she whispers, "but the boy he bit had it coming. He was just awful. But don't *ever* tell Cooper I said that."

We laugh with relief.

Around this time, we begin to think about having a second child. This time our plan is that Tanya will get pregnant. We choose the same donor so our children will have a biological connection, and Tanya is inseminated five or six times. None result in a pregnancy. We suspect there might be a medical issue and discover that she has endometriosis, which the gynecologist thinks is interfering with pregnancy. The doctor operates to clear out the endometriosis and tells Tanya, "Get pregnant now if you're going to do it. The endometriosis will probably come back."

We talk at length about whether to proceed. We've been through so much with my cancer and raising Cooper, who's now five. Given everything, we worry about bringing another baby into this world. We're both ambivalent. Finally, Tanya makes an appointment with Betsy, a healer I worked with when I had cancer. Tanya told Betsy she needed to make a decision about having a second child and that she only intended to come for one appointment. This limit is typical Tanya. Don't process too long; just make a decision and move on.

As Tanya would later tell it, she lay down on the couch, relaxed, went into a trancelike state during a guided meditation. In that state, it was clear that she didn't want to proceed with more inseminations.

I hadn't realized how worried I was about having another child, but when Tanya comes home and announces her decision, I feel hugely relieved.

And as time passes, we never regret our choice.

SPIDERS IN THE CORNER

In both of my cancer experiences, there's been a spiritual aspect to my healing. The first time, just after Cooper was born in 1986, I'd been disconnected from anything spiritual for years. I'd left Mendocino County and moved to San Francisco, gone to law school, and honed the rational part of my brain. Reconnecting to my spiritual and emotional aspects was integral to my recovery.

At that time, my Uncle Bill from my father's hometown in Georgia took on my healing as a personal quest. Every day he wrote a prayer on a small scrap of paper. Once a week, he hand-addressed an envelope to me and stuffed it with the prayers for the week. Even though I knew he was dedicated to what I considered a rather fringy form of Christianity, I cherished every letter he sent and saved them all.

I'm open to many forms of spiritual healing. This view led me to Healing Man, to use the holy water from Lourdes that my neighbor gave me, and to collect healing sand from the small church in Taos, New Mexico. Now, a year and a half after my original diagnosis, it has led Tanya and me to Nevada County in the Sierra foothills. I've just finished chemotherapy and I'm trying to heal from all the treatments.

Tanya and I walk onto an open-air porch on a house hanging over a deep ravine. The air smells of incense and the dry grass of midsummer. The Yuba River runs clear and cold below.

Twenty-five other people are gathered around a small Nepalese woman who sits in lotus position. Her hair is pulled back into a bun.

She wears traditional Nepali clothing. Before her is a basket of rice grains. She chants, yawns, chants some more, and looks at her palm as if she's reading it.

Next to her is a young Nepalese man, perhaps twenty-five. He wears a traditional hat and long shirt and American-style cargo pants. He frowns a little, his expression serious.

On her other side sits an American woman with long graying hair. She gets up to greet us. "I'm Andi," she says. "There's no order to things. Just come up when you're ready."

We're on this mountaintop outside Grass Valley, California, to see a healer named Aama Bambo, whom I learned about from my last mediation client, himself a Buddhist teacher and shaman. He told me that Aama is the most powerful healer he's ever worked with.

After nineteen months of grappling with cancer, it seems worth a try.

One at a time, people from the group approach Aama and tell her their problem. The rest of us sit quietly and listen. Each person sits on the zabuton in front of Aama and tells Pramad, the interpreter, about a problem—such things as arthritis, sore shoulders, suicidal thoughts, stomach ailments. Aama prescribes remedies: meditation, prayers, massage with mustard seed oil, detailed rituals. She prays, throws grains of rice, touches the body with a small brush, a knife, another holy object made of metal. She anoints foreheads with ash. When she's done with each person, she lifts her hands in prayer to signify the healing is over.

After I watch her work with four or five people, I go up and sit before her, bow, and tell her my story: tongue cancer, three surgeries on my neck and tongue, seven weeks of radiation, and four months of chemotherapy. She chants and says, through Pramad, "This is karma. You're in the hands of the gods." She says that the medicines I have taken have made me much better, but I'm not completely healed. I need to pray to Tara. White Tara. The goddess of compassion, long life, and healing. She gives me a piece of tin foil, into which she's put rice grains and ash. "Pray. Then eat seven grains of rice, anoint your forehead with the ash, and rub the ash on your neck. Do this every morning until it runs out." Then she says she wants to see me two more times during this retreat, and I recognize that she thinks my condition is serious. Nobody else has been told to come back.

When it's Tanya's turn, Aama tells her to pray to Medicine Buddha and Green Tara, the feisty goddess of peace and protection.

The next day, another group waits to see Aama on the porch. I have session two with her. She looks at me intently and says I'm getting better. More chants, more prayers, holy water in my mouth and sprinkled on my head.

Tears pour down my cheeks. Aama brushes my face, pats the top of my head, my shoulders, my neck, my back, and finishes by anointing my forehead and neck with ash.

On day three, we meet on the porch again. This time Aama doesn't speak to me at all; when I sit down, she begins praying and chanting.

Back home, we realize we don't know a *thing* about praying to Tara—green or white—or Medicine Buddha. Until we can talk to Andi, we have to make up our own ritual. I have a small Tara statue and a Medicine Buddha postcard that a friend gave me when I was first diagnosed. We set these on a monkey pod table that my father made in 1949 just after I was born. We add a ceramic sculpture of a female figure wearing a necklace that I made in the 1990s, a stone heart that Tanya gave me last year, and a small stone sculpture of an angel that my brother Whit and his wife Mary gave us many years ago. We light incense and candles, meditate, and pray.

A few days later, in the space of less than a week, I start getting cards and emails from my cousins in Georgia, the children of my Uncle Bill who sent the prayers to me in 1986. I can't imagine what's going on. I've been fighting this cancer for nineteen months, so why the cards and emails now?

I call my brother Whit to ask him about it. "Could it be that Mother didn't tell our cousins what's been going on with me?" My mother is the family communicator, the central hub. She's always on the phone with someone, including my cousins. As the last elder of her generation, she's the person they turn to. In fact, my cousins aren't even in my address book on my computer. Between family reunions, they communicate with my mother about our family.

"Next time you talk to her," Whit says, "just casually ask her."

A few days later, the phone rings; caller ID indicates that it's my mother.

"Yo, Mom," I say. "How are you?"

"WONDERFUL." She updates me on all the family news.

"I'm getting all these sweet get-well cards and emails from the Georgia cousins," I say. "It sounds like they didn't know that I was sick until now. Didn't you tell them?"

My mother hems and haws, making excuses like: "I didn't know if you would want me to tell them" and "I didn't want them to bother you."

"What in the world would make you think that they would *bother* me?" I ask, getting agitated. "They've always been *completely* appropriate. All they're doing is sending get well cards and emails!"

"Well, I didn't really know what was going on," she says.

"Mother, you've known about everything *every* single step of the way," I say, completely bewildered. "We called you all the time to update you. What do you *mean* you didn't know?"

And then my mother gets vague. Nothing she says makes any sense. I'm completely astounded by this conversation. About to cry, I make an excuse to hang up, and the next thing I know I'm crying uncontrollably. I can't believe that my mother didn't tell my cousins that I've been sick, that even today the doctors still think I'm terminal.

It's not that my cancer is too traumatic for her to talk about; everyone in her retirement community knows about my illness, and she constantly gives me messages from them. On most Sundays, she calls me to check in, so that she can give a report about how I'm doing to everyone at her lunch table. Her friends all over the world know.

I get in a hot shower and continue crying. Tanya tries to comfort me, but I'm inconsolable. I feel like a motherless child.

After my shower, I call my brother Warren because my mother mentioned that he had talked to my cousins. Warren says that our cousin Marilyn called him because she'd felt uncomfortable after talking to my mother on the phone. She wanted to know if I was okay. He told her I had serious cancer and that he "guessed it would be okay" to tell my other cousins, but they shouldn't "inundate" me with cards and emails.

When he learns I've gotten two cards and one email, he's actually angry and wants to call Marilyn to tell her he isn't pleased!

"Don't call her!" I beg him. "What's *wrong* with you? Why are you upset that I'm getting cards?"

"Mother was just respecting your privacy," Warren says. "There's no reason to be upset."

And here we are again, in completely familiar territory: Somehow, I'm the problem. Once again, we're mired in our family dynamic, although it's been quite a while since it last erupted. I thought I was beyond being hurt by my family anymore. In fact, I'm disturbed that I'm sunk deep in this dark place again. Aren't you supposed to grow up and get over this stuff? I'm sixty years old, for God's sake!

I try to dream up an explanation, any explanation, for my mother's behavior. Is my mother afraid that I'll get the attention that she wants for herself? Does she think my cousins don't matter? Is it related to her judgments about the South? Did she simply think it wasn't important enough to mention? Did she forget?

I call Ann. "I need a consultation. A reality check." I tell her the simple facts without embellishing them with how I feel. "Is it weird that my cousins have just *now* found out that I have cancer?"

"I can't imagine talking to anyone close to me and not having what's going on with you be one of the important topics," she tells me. "All my friends and family know. They ask about you each time we talk." She can tell I'm upset. "Should I come over?"

"No, I'll be fine. I just needed someone besides Tanya to tell me I'm not crazy to have feelings about this."

But the feelings linger.

A few days later on a gray, foggy morning in early August, I sit at the kitchen table with my laptop, feeling gray myself as I ponder my family of origin.

With the exception of one orange dahlia that waves in the wind on the deck, the colors outside are gray and green: gray sky, gray wooden deck, gray umbrella; gray glass table; deep green redwood tree, bright green apple tree, crayon-green wisteria vines, dark green magnolia tree.

My mind grasps at wisps of memories. I simply can't understand what happened.

The phone interrupts my musings about my family. Andi, the woman who organized everything for Aama Bombo, is calling to check in. She gives us mantras to chant when we're meditating. "Do it out loud," she says. "It's more powerful that way." Mine is simple, one long sound. Tanya has two mantras, one for Medicine Buddha and one for Green Tara, each with many words.

"My mantra is drooling mantra," Tanya laughs after she hangs up.

"What do you mean?" I ask.

"There are so many words that I'm drooling all over myself," she says by way of explaining her joke. Now she's really tickled. "Drooling mantra. It's not fair. You get one pretty word, and I get all this hard work."

"Yeah, but you only have to do it in the morning," I say. "And I have to do it morning *and* evening."

The next day I'm having breakfast with Ann. "I really don't know how to think about what's going on with my family," I say. "It's often so subtle. And as you know, everything looks so good on the surface."

"It's like those nice men we used to have in our lives," she says. "They always looked so sweet and good to everyone else, and we looked like raging bitches. When, in fact, there were spiders lurking in the corners that nobody but us could see. That's how your family is. All this underlying rage, your dad an alcoholic, your mother saying everything is *wonderful,* your brothers being nice, and you talking about the stinking spider in the room. They always think you're the crazy one."

"Yeah, but understanding it is almost impossible for me."

ANOTHER TRIP SOUTH

"It's one thing to take Cooper to Texas when he's a baby," I say to Tanya shortly after we return from our trip there when he's ten months old. "But I don't want you to take him when he's older unless you're sure you can stand up to any racist or sexist or homophobic comments that people make in front of him. Because you *know* they'll do it."

Tanya doesn't say anything.

But she takes in my message. She goes back every year to see her father, Celestine, her sister, and her nieces and nephews, but she doesn't take Cooper until 1997, when he's eleven. They go to Beaumont alone and I'm not invited. I take them to the airport and relish an empty house, long bubble baths, reading whenever I want to, and eating yogurt and granola for dinner.

Upon their return a week later, Tanya regales anyone and everyone who will listen with Texas stories. "So, we're at my sister's house," she says in her Texas twang. "Her husband, Joe, takes Cooper outside to throw a baseball. Cooper catches the ball and throws it back to Joe and Joe yells, 'Hell, Cooper, you throw the ball like a goddamn girl.' Cooper looks at me and says, 'What's wrong with that, Mom?' and I tell him I haven't a clue."

I'm proud that my son thinks girls are just as good as boys—and relieved I live in a place that fosters this belief.

"Then, we go to my father's house," Tanya continues. "His wife is a born-again Christian, and he's a plain old Southern Baptist. They say a blessing before *every* meal, which y'all know we don't do. But, Cooper's gone to a Jewish summer camp since he was four or five, and I decide to be proactive. Martina's instructions. I tell Daddy that Cooper will bless the meal. Cooper sings the Hebrew song he learned at Jewish summer camp. Daddy says, 'What's that, Cooper?' And Cooper says, 'It's Jewish. My moms aren't Jewish, but the man who gave the sperm so they could have me is Jewish and that makes me part-Jewish.'

"I can promise you, the word sperm has never been uttered in front of my father in his whole life. Nobody at the table said another word. We just ate in silence."

I sigh with relief that I stayed home, grateful that Tanya handled everything.

Still, it's painful to both of us that we aren't accepted by most of her family. Each trip there brings new, painful revelations.

When Celestine died a few years before this trip, Tanya found every single photo of Cooper that we'd ever sent her buried in her bottom drawer under her negligee.

During that same trip, Tanya mentioned Cooper to her cousin. "Who's Cooper?" her cousin asked.

"My son!" Tanya said.

Her cousin turned to Tanya's father. "Have you met him?"

"No," Nelson lied.

Tanya pulled out photographs of our sweet boy and then turned the conversation to her cousin's children.

And years later, in the early 2000s, out of the blue, Tanya's father will call Tanya from Texas. "I just wanted to let you know that Jo and I went to the polls today to vote against gay marriage."

When the time comes for our own gay marriage, Tanya doesn't invite them.

THE LAP OF THE FAMILY

It's the fall of 2009, a few months after my last chemo treatment. Tanya is hammering in the backyard on one of her projects while I relax on the deck. As part of my fall garden prep, I've just pruned the wisteria and cut five of the last incredible dahlias and arranged them in three little vases on the kitchen table: a small, creamy one; two bright yellow ones, six inches across; and two orange, spidery Ms. McKissick dahlias. Ms. McKissick lived over one of our back fences when we moved here in 1986. When she died about fifteen years ago, another neighbor, Renate, rescued some of Ms. McKissick's famous dahlia bulbs so her legacy would live on. This year we've had eight lovely blooms so far.

My mind drifts back to when Cooper was a baby. We'd take him out on the deck to say goodnight most nights. "Good night, moon. Good night, stars. Good night, Ms. McKissick. Good night, Renate." It was our version of goodnight prayers.

The sun beats down on my uncovered head. Little fuzzy gray hairs are sprouting out like a halo. Tanya comes up on the deck and kisses the top of my head. We take a break.

"Are you noticing anything from doing your meditation?" I ask.

"I'm happy. Really happy. And I like puttering and doing all my little projects," she says.

"I think I'm better," I say. "I'm just not worrying so much."

—

Sometime back in June or July, when we were thinking about chemotherapy coming to an end and having some freedom from weekly
infusions, Cooper said he wanted to go on a family vacation. Tanya
and I thought Hawaii. Cooper suggested Calistoga, where we used to
take annual vacations to decompress after Christmas. It's been years
since we've been there with Cooper.

As we drive into Napa Valley, I realize that it's not only the fortieth anniversary of Woodstock; it's the fortieth anniversary of my first
trip to the Roman Spa, which I discovered with David in 1969.

"The town seems smaller," Cooper says as we cruise down
Washington Street. "But I think it's because I'm bigger."

"I remember going back to Winona," Tanya says, referring to her
childhood home in Texas. "As a child, I thought my grandparents'
house was enormous. I was shocked as an adult to see that it was just
a two-bedroom place."

"When I was pregnant with you," I tell Cooper, "Tanya and I went
back to Japan." Tanya and I refer to each other by our first names
when we talk to Cooper, even though he refers to both of us as Mom.
I explain that in my mind, my house in Sasebo was palatial, with
a luscious Japanese garden. It was incredibly disappointing to find
that it was actually a funky beige military house with a tiny concrete
fishpond.

As we walk into our room at the spa, Cooper says, "Nothing has
changed." He's delighted. "It looks just like it always has." Even when
the owners remodeled, they kept the same '50s look. That's what we
like about the place.

We're in the mineral tub that's the size of a small swimming pool
when a young woman comes over to me and says, "Can I ask you a
question?"

"Sure."

"Are you in therapy?" I know she's referring to chemotherapy because she's looking at the scarf on my head.

"I just finished a month ago."

"I had mega chemo," she says. "I was in bed for over a year. That was over seven years ago." She's smiling.

"Good for you," I say, knowing that seven years free of cancer has great meaning.

"Be strong," she says.

In the morning, Tanya wants to go to the park to meditate while Cooper sleeps. We find a spot by the elementary school. Tanya walks and chants in the sun. I sit on a cold metal bench under a redwood tree where I can almost taste the greenness of the fresh-cut grass. I'm done first and find a bench in the sun. The air is clean, electric, like after a rainstorm. Water from an early-morning sprinkling covers my sandals. I stick my feet in the sun to warm up and dry off. I watch an ant walk across the pavement. A Latina woman with a young child walks by. "Good morning," I say. She smiles and says, "Hola."

Later in the day, Cooper, Tanya, and I wander through Calistoga, looking in the shops, and end up at the bookstore, where Cooper spends a long afternoon by himself after Tanya and I stroll back to our hotel. He returns with four books. One is about life after death by Deepak Chopra, which he thinks I might like. One is about end-of-life care, which he thinks he and Tanya should read. One is about finances. I'm a bit startled.

"Are you preparing for me to die?"

"No," he says. "The titles are weird, but if you read the covers, you'll like them. It's stuff we all need to know about."

He starts into the financial book. "What about social security?" he asks. "Tell me how that works."

"You shouldn't count on it when you're planning your future," I say. "The Republicans are always trying to end it."

"Who do they want to give them their Starbucks in the morning or their Subway sandwiches at lunch?" he asks. He's done the math and knows these workers don't make enough to save for retirement. They can barely survive.

We talk about psychological things, about how we raised him. He thinks we were over-involved, controlling, and anxious parents, and that he tried to be "good" to keep us calm. It's ended up being a problem for him, he says.

I think about how hard Tanya and I have worked at being good parents. And here we are with a great kid who still has complaints about us. A part of me is glad he's talking about it and a part of me feels misunderstood.

While we are in Calistoga, I (mostly) put my problems with my mother and brothers out of my mind. But we return home to a long email from my brother Whit, who writes that he's taken on the task of sorting out our family situation and concluded that our mother was simply being respectful of my privacy.

To respond or not? I mentally note that I hadn't been interviewed during his investigation. Tanya says to leave it alone, that I'll never get any satisfaction from trying to communicate about this incident.

"I can't," I say, even though I suspect she's right. "I don't want to bite my tongue anymore."

I find my laptop and write a response, which Tanya edits. Then we work together to make a third draft that we both agree upon. I tell my brothers that I don't see this incident the way they do; that when my feelings are hurt, it makes things worse for me when they work so hard to find an explanation that almost always seems to conclude that I'm the problem.

I feel raw, like someone took an eggbeater to my insides.

That afternoon, Tanya and I walk up to a café in our neighborhood and sit outside in the sun for afternoon tea. I think the British have it right. Such a lovely ritual. A woman and five blond children between four and seven walk by. The kids chatter. One is barefoot and skips along the sidewalk as if she's in a green meadow in the spring. A homeless woman sits at the next table, resting and drinking coffee.

"I'm so stirred up," I say as we begin to walk home. "I feel insecure and unsure of myself." This business with my family feels horrible. This is not my usual way of being. Normally, I'm fairly self-assured.

Tanya's quiet a moment. "Have I told you lately that I love you?" she asks.

I'm suddenly in tears. "I'm not a bad person, am I?"

She steers me over to the edge of the sidewalk, so we don't block foot traffic, and wraps her arms around me.

Several days go by and neither of my brothers responds to my email, although they promptly respond to other emails related to non-controversial family business. I'm disappointed, but not surprised.

I wake up one morning later that week churning with memories. Tanya's in the next room, chanting her meditation. The smell of incense wafts into the bedroom. I pull up the blanket and let my mind drift. The memories, the family drama, and the meditation have stirred me up. I'm wide open, so unsure of myself. What's true?

I ponder the way my family communicates—or fails to communicate. But, like so many problems in my family, this episode will simply be "forgotten." In fact, it's never mentioned again. And in the end I never make sense of it.

CRYSTALLINE DAYS

Tanya and I have been housesitting Dana's houseboat in Sausalito. Seagulls circle, squawking and nose-diving into the bay. An occasional seal peeks out of the water. The salt air feels like home; I've always lived near the ocean.

I'm watering Dana's herb garden on the deck before we leave for Stanford again, feeling both good and nervous. It will be my first appointment since I stopped chemo. What will Dr. Colevas say? Will the cancer be back?

We pile our luggage into shopping carts and wheel them down the wooden pier. Clackety-clack, clickety-clack.

Tanya drives us across the Golden Gate Bridge. Wind whips over the span; August tourists, dressed in shorts and sleeveless tank tops, look frozen. I know this route through San Francisco like the back of my hand. All through law school I drove into the city from Mendocino County along this route. I'd peel off at 19th Avenue to get to my flat with Susan at 22nd and Irving or drive down Lombard to Divisadero when I lived in the Castro. Today, we drive through the city on 19th Avenue and down the Peninsula on I-280. As we get farther south, the fog disappears. My mood soars with more light.

Once we're at the clinic, we don't have to wait long. Dr. Colevas walks into the examining room and shakes my hand. "I want to look at you first. How are you?"

"Good," I say.

He pokes and prods. Another doctor comes in and Dr. Colevas challenges him to find the spots where the original tumors were. He finds nothing.

We discuss alternative treatments and drug trials at UC Davis, Stanford, and back East. "The problem is that you don't qualify. You've got to have tumors to qualify. Otherwise, how do we know the drugs are working?"

"I can think of worse problems to have," I say.

"Just to be clear," he says. "If something comes back, I'd treat you the same way we did before. We know it works. And in the meantime, I think you should continue the honeymoon and do nothing."

"When should I come back?"

"Two to three months, your choice. But if anything changes, I want to hear about it right away," he says.

And that's that. Another reprieve. Is this an answer to my prayers or just a temporary honeymoon? Who knows?

I'm in the hands of the gods.

A week later, I'm in a sunny conference room in a beautiful, modern building on Fifth Street in Berkeley, accompanying my mother to her appointment with her lawyer because she needs to revise her will and medical forms.

"I changed your son Whit's name from Grady Whitfield Reaves to Whitfield Reaves, which he requested," the lawyer tells her.

"That's fine," my mother says. "I'd like Marti's name to be Ellen Martin Reaves, but she says that's not right."

"It's not my legal name anymore, Mom." This is the third time she's raised the issue of my name. I'm trying to be patient with her each time, but it's wearing thin.

"I don't like it," my mother had announced after David and I returned to the States from Mexico and I told her my new name. "It sounds like martini."

"Sorry, Mom. You can still call me Marti."

My social security card continued to say Martin Reaves Patton until this year when I went to the funky office in downtown Berkeley to apply for social security disability. There I was, post-9/11, with a driver's license that said Martina Ellen Reaves, a birth certificate that said Ellen Martin Reaves, and records with Social Security that said Martin Reaves Patton. I had to dig out my divorce papers from 1981, and now, I'm the proud owner of a Social Security card that says Martina Ellen Reaves.

A few days after the visit to the lawyer, Tanya and I do our new morning ritual: she gets up, showers, and starts her chanting meditation. I get up, shower, and start mine when she finishes hers.

"Wanna walk to Fat Apple's and get a bran muffin?" she asks when I'm done. "Or do you want to eat here?"

"Fat Apple's," I say.

I look at our poodle, Mollie. "Want to go for a walk?" She can't believe her good fortune. Long walks aren't usually part of the morning regimen. She went to the groomer two days ago and looks fluffy and beautiful, with a new bandanna around her neck. She prances to the front door.

We pass by our neighbors' dahlia garden, which fills their front yard. Some stalks are over five feet tall. We pass the new construction on the corner, where the family of four is adding two bedrooms. Wandering down Josephine Street, we check out gardens and house additions. When we arrive at Fat Apple's, I get the muffins and drinks to go so we can sit in the sun with Mollie. Margot, a long-time waitress there, comes outside to sit with us.

"How *are* you?" she asks me. We used to be regulars at Fat Apple's, but since my diagnosis, we have been coming less frequently.

"I'm really fine. I finished chemotherapy a month and a half ago," I say. "They can't find any cancer. But, of course, they think it will come back."

"You look great," she says, putting her hand on my arm.

Other workers come out to say hello, Jessica, Corazón. Janet is pregnant, less than a month from her due date, glowing, full, ready to pop.

As we approach Tanya's fifty-sixth birthday in late August, she announces that all she wants is to go to our cabin on the Russian River with me and Cooper. He takes two days off work and she gets her wish.

Recent vacations with Cooper have been lovely, both to our cabin and to Calistoga. But now we're all gritchy. The three of us aren't meshing. Late in the afternoon of the first full day we decide to go to Goat Rock Beach. I'm drinking my Chinese herbs as Cooper drives us down the country road. "Please slow down," I say. He's immediately annoyed. "It's not about your driving," I say. "It's about me spilling my herbs."

He drives along the road to the beach and reaches a spot where he has to go left or right. To the right is a lovely expanse of white sand leading up to the mouth of the Russian River. There, the bright red ball of a sun hovers over a thick, low fog bank. To the left in the shade, rocky, wild cliffs rise over a small beach with crashing waves.

"Which way should I go?" Cooper asks.

"Right," Tanya and I say in unison.

He goes *left!* I'm incredulous. Grinding my teeth, I ask, "Why would you ask us which way we want to go and then go the other way?"

"Because the cliffs are so beautiful on this side," he says.

We get out of the car, but there's no sun on the cliff side. It's windy, dark, and cold. "I want to go to the sunny side," I say.

Tanya and I walk toward the long, sunny beach, but there's a huge rock blocking the way with two paths around it. I head to the route above the rock. But Cooper heads toward the water, where the second route passes between the ocean and the rock. The tide is coming in; enormous waves pound the beach and crash onto the rock, then churn and grind back out, briefly leaving a sandy walkway before the next huge wave curls over. I look up and see a sign that says: "This is one of the most dangerous beaches in California. Sleeper waves will surprise you. Don't take your eyes off the water."

Tanya and I both yell into the wind, "This way!"

"I want to go *this* way!" he yells back.

"Look at the sign!" I scream, pointing. He keeps walking toward the water, and then all hell breaks loose.

We're all shrieking at once, and Cooper finally shouts, "I'm twenty-three! I can decide which way to go! Quit being overprotective."

"It's my birthday!" Tanya screams. "And I don't want to watch you get sucked out to sea. Look at the fucking sign!"

I'm livid. I rarely give up in family fights; I'll keep trying to work things out longer than is reasonable. But I'm just *done*. I have no reserves, no stamina. I walk over to Cooper, take the car keys from him, and walk up to the car. He and Tanya follow. We get in and I drive back toward the cabin.

"Come on," Cooper says quietly. "Can't we just walk on the beach?"

"We can," I say, "but it's gonna take me a while to cool down. So this won't be the relaxed walk on the beach that we were planning."

I drive down to the sunny beach. We walk separately toward the mouth of the river. I'm near tears. Other families can come to the beach and have a good time together. What's our problem? Are we fighting because it's safe to do it now that I'm better? I pick up small rocks that appeal to me: a gray one with a white band on it, a smooth black one. The sun is enormous, glowing red behind the fog now, slowly sinking toward the ocean. Just before it sets, the three of us walk back to the car and return to our cabin in silence.

Slowly, everything calms down. We don't talk about our fight. We eat dinner and relax. Late that night, after Tanya has gone to bed, Cooper and I end up in a conversation about the line between hope and acceptance when it comes to medical matters such as mine. He's reading the book he got on our Calistoga vacation about end-of-life issues. The author says that people can be optimistic too long, feeling like they have to do it for their family. Cooper wonders when hope becomes denial.

"Do you think I'm in denial?" I ask him.

"No, I don't," he says. "You seem good now." But he's confused about when to hold on to hope and when to give up.

I don't have answers, but I try. "I believe you can have hope until the very end," I say, "and at the same time accept that you're dying. It doesn't have to be one or the other. It can be both." I can see his brain working to absorb this idea, and I know that he could go on talking, but I'm exhausted. I have to meditate and go to sleep.

We say goodnight, on good terms again, and as I meditate, I reflect on the contrasts of the day. Could we have had this last conversation without the fight that preceded it?

In September, I decide that I'm strong enough to return to a dance class with Tanya. Before my diagnosis, we took lots of lessons: West Coast swing, East Coast swing, rumba, cha cha. While I've been sick, Tanya's classes have kept her sane and given her a reprieve from caretaking.

I'm joining a rumba class and today we're taking a private lesson to prepare me for it. Ooh la la, it's a slinky dance. We practice our Cuban motion, watching ourselves in the mirrors that cover the walls of the studio. Our teacher, Kate, says, "No white girl motion, ladies.

No prancing." Unfortunately, we're white as magnolia blossoms and our motion is not the best, but we improve quickly. As Tanya leads me around the floor, I tear up, thinking how long it's been since we danced like this.

In the car on the way home from class, I tell her about the new airline check-in procedures: you can get your ticket with a barcode sent to your cell phone and use it to check in.

"This is really bad. I can't do anything with my phone," I say. "One of the things I thought was great when I first got cancer was that I wouldn't have to learn all this new technology."

"Don't think that way," Tanya laughs. "I don't want you to have any incentive not to go on living."

On a warm morning in early September, Tanya and I return to the hillside outside Grass Valley to see Aama Bombo. The hills are covered with dry, yellow grasses; the sky, cloudless.

We arrive at Andi's house on time and wander into the living room. Aama Bombo walks in, sees us, and smiles. It's rare to see this joyful face; when she's working, she's always somber. Pramad, her interpreter, comes in and hugs us. I'm surprised. In the month since we last saw them, they've seen hundreds of people with multitudes of problems. I didn't expect to be remembered.

The session starts. People sit in chairs and on the floor of the porch, respectfully waiting for their turn to speak with Aama. This time, she begins with a little teaching. She shows us the tools that she uses in her healing, some of which are over a hundred years old, used by her father before her. Pramad translates as Aama talks. She describes her father as a great healer and says she learned from him.

Then Aama asks people to come forward and tell her their problems. She deals with a man who was sexually abused as a child; a man who struggles with dark thoughts; a woman long past menopause who gets so hot each night that sweat soaks through a thick comforter.

When it's my turn, I sit before her, cross-legged on a zabuton. She's in lotus position. I tell her that I have meditated every morning and every evening since I last saw her a month ago; that I had trouble with my family of origin; that I worry less and less all the time; and that I want to know what else she thinks I should be doing.

"Nom?" she says. By now, I know this means, what's my name?

The thought crosses my mind to say "Marti" rather than "Martina" and I wonder what difference it would make in how she responds. But Pramad says, "Martina." She starts chanting and pointing her thumb to spots on her palm. Then she begins talking, and Pramad translates. Things are better. The medicines I'm taking are working. I should keep praying the way I am praying, every day.

Then she prescribes a detailed ritual she wants me to do. On a Friday in November, I should make a clay figure of myself, adorn her, put her on a tray with nine kinds of beans and many flowers, and leave the tray outside overnight. On Saturday night after 9 p.m., I should take the tray to the top of a hill, pray, and leave it to disintegrate with the elements. I'll then enter a new phase.

An odd prescription, I think, and nothing like what she's prescribed for others, but I'm ready for a ritual of transition.

Back in Berkeley, I notice all the signs of change: Yesterday, I didn't have to paint my eyebrows on. Tiny dark eyebrows are growing back. The hair on my head is about an inch long, with fuzzy longer gray hairs and shorter dark brown hairs. I decide it's time for grooming and go to Solano Avenue to get my hair done and my eyebrows and chin waxed. It seems utterly unfair to me that the hair on my head fell out but not the hair on my chin.

I just want my hair buzzed down to half an inch and my ears and neckline cleaned up so it can grow in evenly. I walk into one of those fourteen-dollars-a-cut places and try to explain the situation to an Asian woman who smiles sweetly but doesn't appear to understand what I'm saying. Finally, I pull off my hat, gesture a half-inch with my fingers, and she motions me to sit in the chair. Buzz, buzz, buzz. "Sexy," she pronounces. I think she's nuts, but I'm smiling because the little hairlets do look pretty cute now.

I drive up the street and find that Joi, the place I usually go to for girl stuff like waxing and nails, is booked until Saturday, so I go to the yuppie place across the street which has an opening right now. I lie on a massage table as Carrie methodically removes eyebrow and chin hairs I don't need. Wax, press the cloth, pull, sting. Despite the sensations, I'm zoned out and completely relaxed when I leave.

Now what? I want a bath, but I decide what I "should" do is buy my Chinese herbs, which are almost gone. Ah, the farmers' market is happening. I buy four gorgeous O'Henry peaches that cost a whopping $7.50. This is completely absurd, I think, but I buy them anyway. Summer squash, black beans, green beans, salsa and guacamole, and I'm set for dinner.

At home, I sink into a bubble bath while Tanya cooks the squash with onions.

The sun behind me beats down on my bare head and neck, warming me all the way to my toes, which are wet in my sandals from watering the garden. A half moon floats in the blue sky in front of me.

Even if I didn't know the date, I'd know that it's fall. There are spiders everywhere. The redwood tree is dropping bits of detritus all over the backyard. The cherry tomato plants are looking scraggly and the leaves are moldy. But the biggest sign is the light, the crispness of the sun in Northern California in the fall.

Healing Man says, "When you feel the sun, remember it has travelled 92 million miles, just for you." I'm remembering and soaking every bit into my body. I change position and the sun shines down on my face. My eyes are closed and I see red, a bright vibrant red, and my lashes and the sun glinting off the frames of my glasses. My washing machine whooshes and the saws of the workers next door grind. I throw my head back so the sun can reach my neck. The scar from my surgeries stretches. My neck crinkles. Everything feels fine.

FAMILY TROUBLES

Cooper's smart. Charming. Honest. Creative. Artistic. But by the end of fifth grade in 1997, he's diagnosed with learning differences, a mix of auditory processing deficits and dyslexia. These issues aren't easily defined and they don't fit into the usual categories. As his hormones kick in, other traits arise that often go hand-in-hand with different learning styles: He's self-conscious and insecure. The person who tests him suggests that he'd do better in small classes, with "hands on" learning and individual attention. We are avid proponents of public school. When many people we know sent their children to private schools starting at kindergarten, we intentionally chose our local public school. The public middle school is only half a block from our house and we always assumed he'd go there. Reluctantly, we enroll him in the East Bay School for the Arts for grades six through eight, where he produces paintings, sculptures, ceramics, and woodcarvings that fill our walls and, when we run out of space, our attic. He's engaged and prolific. This school was made for him.

He's also dogged about addressing his learning issues and spends several summers learning to read faster, write better, speak more effectively. Seldom complaining, he analyzes what's wrong and works on it. By the fall of eighth grade, in 1999, we start to think about high school. Cooper's middle school was perfect for him; high school is not so simple. The educational consultant recommends against Berkeley High and we begin to visit private high schools.

—

I'm home alone for a brief moment, getting dressed to visit one of the high schools while Tanya picks up Cooper from a sleepover at Anthony's house. The phone rings.

"There's a woman in a car accident repeating this phone number," a voice says. There's a pause. Adrenaline surges through my body.

"She's okay."

"Where?"

"MLK and Vine." Right by Anthony's house.

"Tell her I'm coming."

I race to my car and hear sirens screaming as I drive down MLK. The ambulance arrives at the same moment I pull into the bus stop on the corner. I look up the street. Our Volvo wagon is skewed sideways in the street, the driver's side completely smashed in, windows shattered. A huge, oversized pickup truck is stopped beside the car; the driver, disheveled, in a stupor, leans against the fender. Cooper, his friends, and many strangers are circled around the wreckage. Traffic is stopped in both directions.

I run to the driver's side and peer through the shattered glass window. The door won't open. I run around to the passenger side and a man sitting with Tanya moves out so I can get in.

Tanya is frozen in her seat, teeth gritted, hand gripped on the emergency brake.

"I'm here," I say softly. She doesn't move or say a word. I reach for her hand, but she's rigid, unmoving, silent. There's no blood.

A paramedic asks me to get out of the car and climbs in to talk with her. Eventually, they pull her out from the passenger side of the car and put her on a stretcher and into the ambulance to take her to the hospital. I'm grateful that they say I can ride along. In some places, only a legal spouse would be able to accompany her. I quickly make arrangements with Anthony's mother for Cooper to stay with her and climb in the ambulance.

At Alta Bates Emergency Room, doctors examine her and ask five thousand questions. Tanya seems rattled, but okay, they think. The accident seems to have been an enormous fender bender, but nothing more, and she doesn't even stay overnight. We pick up Cooper from his friend's house and settle in at home. For the rest of the weekend, Tanya lies on the living room floor in front of the fireplace, sore and achy, but apparently fine.

Monday morning, we trudge up the metal stairs to the second floor of the loft where we both have our businesses. Tanya loves her work. She thrives on it. She specializes in legal malpractice, suing lawyers on behalf of their clients when the lawyers have gouged them for fees or done a bad job. There's always plenty of work, unfortunately, because there are a lot of incompetent or outright dishonest lawyers out there. She's at the peak of her career, known throughout the country for her work. She's just written a book with some of her colleagues about attorney misconduct and is often called as an expert witness in cases involving malpractice.

She's one of the few lawyers I know who truly enjoys her work.

When we enter her office, I see that it's in its usual state: her eight-foot-long desk has multiple stacks of files; there's an array of material spread out on the floor; files are piled high on the coffee table in front of the gray couch. Files are stacked three feet tall on the floor.

But there's order to this apparent chaos. Tanya always knows what's in every single stack. She can call the office from home and say, "Go into my office. The pile on the right side of my desk on the floor is the Smith case." And then she can tell her assistant to find a particular document in a particular file.

But today, she looks around and bursts into tears. Tanya hardly ever cries, and certainly not at work. She can't figure out what she's supposed to do. She's confused and unable to remember where anything is. I think it's just too soon, that she needs more rest, and I take her back home.

The next day, she goes to see her doctor, who says her damage is very mild. "Your confusion is temporary," he says. "It will pass. Just give it time."

We believe our doctor and do what we need to do to keep Tanya's business intact. I sit with her and go through her cases, figuring out, slowly, where things stand with each one and what has to be done. It's almost like twenty years ago when I was her law clerk. I still know how to help her organize. We postpone what can be postponed and hire other lawyers to do the work that can't wait.

Tanya sees acupuncturists, chiropractors, cranial/sacral specialists. She takes supplements touted to enhance brain function. Months pass. All the while, doctors keep saying she'll get better, just give it time. "After all," they say, "you didn't lose consciousness. It's just a mild traumatic brain injury. You didn't even have a full concussion."

Assuming everything will be fine, we sell our loft in Emeryville and purchase, build-out, and move both of our offices to a small building that is so close to home we can walk to work. For months, Tanya sits in her peaceful, elegant space; the phones get answered; she refers cases to the other lawyers whom she's supervising; she rocks Kim's baby, who comes to work with Kim each day for the first six months.

When her functioning doesn't improve after six months, subtle insinuations begin. You can feel it in the questions people ask—doctors, and even our friends. They're wondering if Tanya has an emotional problem. Maybe she's malingering. They wonder what benefit she gets by not getting better. What's the secondary gain? Could she be doing this to get disability benefits—as if Tanya would rather get disability than do the work she loves! Some people actually make jokes about how their memory is beginning to go and fail to see the distinction between normal aging and what Tanya's going through. She is, after all, just forty-seven.

I'm both bewildered and enraged. On the one hand, I know

Tanya's not doing well. On the other, I can see that it's not that obvious to the casual observer. Even Cooper occasionally asks why she's not back at work.

I begin to find myself ever so slowly having to do things to compensate for Tanya's deficits. I pay more attention to big picture finances. I work harder to earn more money, becoming the primary breadwinner. When she misses something in a conversation, I intervene to smoothly explain it to her. It's all subtle, though, not dramatic, a matter of emphasis.

Cooper ends up at a small private high school in Berkeley and seems to transition well, despite being upset that he isn't at Berkeley High, where all his friends are. The small class size and project-based learning is what he needs most, and that's simply not available at the public school. I feel fortunate to be able to send him there and disappointed that Berkeley High won't work for him.

Meanwhile, we fight with two insurance companies: our disability insurance company and Liberty Mutual, our car insurance company. It's a nightmare. The disability company refuses to categorize Tanya as fully disabled. The adjuster doesn't want to rely on the voluminous reports we've supplied and insists that Tanya see a company-chosen neurologist. Hasn't she been tested, prodded, and analyzed enough already? We're sent to Sacramento to meet with Dr. Brooker. Is it really possible there isn't a competent person closer to home? Annoyed, we comply, knowing it's our job to "cooperate" with our insurance companies.

We expect a sleazy insurance company hack like the other doctors from insurance companies that she's seen, but Dr. Brooker is kind and seems sincere. A little paranoid, I wonder if he's just ingratiating himself to us to see if he can dig up information to help the insurance company. At this point, I don't trust our insurance companies to have our best interests in mind.

Dr. Brooker takes time with Tanya and administers two full days of tests; he interviews me to understand more about her functioning. When it's over, we drive back to Berkeley, unsure what to think.

Weeks later, his report finally arrives at Tanya's doctor's office, but only after we insist that we receive a copy. Even though it's Tanya's life, the report belongs to the insurance company that paid Dr. Brooker, not to Tanya.

We eventually obtain a copy from our doctor. We decide that she doesn't need to read volumes about her impairments. Alone, I read the pages and pages of results, amazed by what the doctor says: Tanya is not malingering; in fact, she would like nothing more than to be okay, to be able to go back to work. The tests confirm that Tanya is telling the truth about her condition: her memory and executive functioning are not working at a high level. And she must have those functions, Dr. Brooker says, to be a litigator.

"Oh, my God," Tanya says when I give her the news. "If the doctor for the *insurance* company thinks I'm impaired, things must be *really* bad."

With Dr. Brooker's report in hand and almost a year after the accident, we meet with our own neurologist to figure out what to do. The examining room is so small that I have to sit behind Tanya, rather than beside her. The doctor explains that Tanya's brain function is impaired, that her memory is affected, and what's worse, she's often completely unaware of the dysfunction. Although her IQ and intelligence are unaffected, her short-term memory and ability to multitask are impaired. She has diminished attention and processing speed; her visual memory, spelling, and reading comprehension are below normal. "There may be some improvement over time," he says, "but the really rapid healing occurs soon after the accident."

Tears well as I listen, and I feel compelled to ask the hard question. "If it were you, doctor, would you continue pouring your savings into the business to try to keep it going? Or, are you trying to tell us that Tanya will have to stop practicing law?"

He hesitates, then looks at Tanya, not me. "You started out at a very high level. It's not likely that you'll regain the brainpower you had before the accident."

Tears flow down my cheeks. Tanya is quiet.

"You need to get to acceptance about what has happened," the doctor says. He refers her to a therapist who specializes in brain injuries. She is gentle as she helps Tanya come to terms with her injury, to grieve the loss of her life's work.

Despite Dr. Brooker's report, there are still complications with the lawyer for the car insurance company, Shelley Kramer, who's insistent that Tanya is lying about her disability. Convinced that Tanya is working when she says she can't, she hires an investigator to conduct surveillance, which we learn about from Bob at the corner liquor store where Tanya buys a Coke every afternoon. "Hey, Tanya," he says one day. "There's a guy in here asking questions about you and slinking around the neighborhood taking videos of you and Martina."

In the legal process, we request copies of the videos, which actually prove that *I'm* the one working. The investigator thinks I'm Tanya because I walk to work with my briefcase, dressed like a lawyer! Tanya tags along beside me in a T-shirt and jeans, looking like a teenager.

Even after this fiasco, Shelley won't settle the case. She insists on taking it all the way to arbitration, a full-blown trial that lasts five days, to try to prove Tanya is able to work. One of her closing arguments is that Tanya still has all her work clothes in her closet and that she'll pull them out and go back to work the minute the trial is over!

We win. Of course. But only if you can call this winning: Liberty Mutual has to pay us policy limits, meaning the total amount available in the insurance contract, which is all we'd asked for from the very beginning. Policy limits don't begin to compensate us for the fact that Tanya can't practice law anymore. After half of the proceeds are paid to our lawyers and other professionals for handling the case, we end up with about what we've spent from savings in the two years since the accident to keep her business afloat, an amount that's probably equivalent to what Shelley's law firm was paid to litigate the case. So, in fact, we lose and the insurance company loses. It paid more money to fight the case than if it had just settled in the first place. Not to mention the many months of our upset and anguish.

With the arbitration over, we *finally* try to move on with life. We both think that we've sheltered Cooper from the worst of this experience and that his life has gone on as normal. Such denial. Of course, we're wrong, and he'll later give us the details of how hard that first year was on him. We plodded through it, one step at a time, profoundly disconnected, without even realizing it.

What's there to say about such an event? That life isn't the same? Eventually, Tanya refers her remaining clients to other lawyers to have their cases completed and closes her office for good. Fortunately, despite her reputation for being an intense, hard-working lawyer, Tanya has *always* had interests beyond her law practice. A naturally joyful person, she has many talents: mothering, nesting, building things, remodeling, gardening, beautifying almost anything, cooking, playing, and, finally, dancing, which is supposed to be good for brain function. She slowly wades back into her life, and after a few years, she's swimming freely. Her life does not end with the accident, but her focus changes dramatically.

UH OH

It's our anniversary, September 14, 2009. One year ago, Tanya and I got married. Since then, the California Supreme Court ruled that our marriage is valid, despite the passage of the anti-gay marriage initiative. No more same-sex couples can marry in the future, but those of us already married have valid marriages.

I'm anxious. With chemo over, a part of me is waiting to see if the cancer will come back. I have two tiny spots on my neck. At my last visit with Dr. Colevas, I pointed them out. "I don't know what they are," he said. "They might be cancer. They might be nothing. They don't show on the scan. We'll just have to watch."

Since then, I've spent many days ignoring them. In fact, there have been stretches of time during which I've felt completely well, in which I've temporarily forgotten that I've had cancer that's supposed to be terminal. These stretches alternate with moments of acute awareness of the spots as I fret in front of the magnifying mirror studying my neck.

Today, one seems different. My agreement with Tanya is that I won't hide things from her, but I realize that I've been doing just that, off and on, because she's already had so much to worry about. I want to protect her, but that's not our deal. I walk into the kitchen. "I have to talk to you," I say. "Come look. I know it's our anniversary, but this is really bothering me."

She puts on her glasses and carefully inspects. "There are definitely two bumps. This one on your neck looks a little bigger. The one under your chin looks a little different."

"Shit, I was afraid you'd say that. I don't *want* this." I'm about to cry. Amazingly calm, Tanya holds me.

We discuss whether to call Dr. Colevas. She's supposed to go to Texas to see her father tomorrow. She missed her annual visits while I was sick and will be gone for four days. I don't want to go to the doctor without her. I want to have four days to write and read and relax. We decide it can wait, that nothing is urgent.

"I'm going to sizzle them away while you're gone."

The remarkable thing about talking to her is that the nausea in the pit of my stomach subsides. We go to lunch at O Chame and eat our favorite meal: corn pancakes, blanched spinach, grilled eel on endive.

At home, we exchange anniversary presents: I give her a small yellow ceramic bowl to hold incense while she meditates in the mornings; she gives me a Tibetan chime to use at the beginning and end of meditations.

Later in the afternoon, Tanya motions me to follow her into the small room off our bedroom where our altar is set up. "Lie down on the couch," she says. I sit. "Down all the way."

She shows me a large Tibetan singing bowl, gently places it on my chest, and hits it with padded mallet. The sound reverberates in the room and vibrates inside my body.

"I decided I could spend my birthday money on anything I wanted, and this is what I wanted. It's going to sit on the bed. If you're scared while I'm gone, lie down and hit it. It will calm you."

I feel transported as I lie on the couch while she taps the bowl.

The next week, the phone rings. "I'm at the airport, ready to get on BART," Tanya says. She's home from Texas. "I'll call you when I get to the MacArthur station."

"Good." I jump up, put on my gym clothes, walk the dog, go to the gym, come home, shower, and I'm ready for the call from MacArthur. That's how cool my gym is, five minutes away and thirty minutes in and out.

I gather her up and see that she's a wreck. More Texas stories. Not the funny kind. She tells me about conversations with the son of her father's wife, who hung around for most of her visit. This was unusual. She usually gets to spend time alone with her father. This time, his wife's son talked nonstop: "I wanted to be a marine biologist, but I went out there to the college and all they have is faggots teaching." Or: "Those N***** football players date the white girls. It's disgusting." Tanya goes on and on and on and on about the conversations until I'm ready to scream, and I realize how horrible it was for her, that she's traumatized.

In a daze, she's sound asleep by early evening.

A week later, I wake up, throw back the clean sheets and comforter. Shower. Fluff my little hairlets, now a half-inch long. Light the incense. Light the candle. Sit on the pillows to meditate. Chant.

My mind romps all over the place. Apparently, I can still multitask after all! I chant, carefully moving forward, bead by bead. But another part of my mind is thinking. Sunlight comes in the top of the shades and reflects off the mirror behind me onto the Tara *thangka* in front of me. There I see, reflected in the glass, the birds on the roof of the house next door. The candle flickers. The smoky smell of incense fills the room. Birds squawk. Kids yell on their way to King Middle School.

Chant on. Rededicate myself to meditating. Brain keeps thinking about breakfast, writing, loving my life.

I feel myself grapple with my situation a bit differently. It's hard to describe. Maybe it's a refinement on having hope and acceptance at the same time. I'm mostly content. I feel strong and healthy and so alive. Yet I'm beginning to accept that this could all come to an abrupt end.

I put off making medical appointments and relish the spaciousness of an empty calendar.

"Okay, check my neck again," I say to Tanya a week later. "I'm not inclined to do anything. I've got the same two bumps I had when I last saw Dr. Colevas. One might be a little different, but not a lot. I don't want to call him unless you think I should."

She puts on her glasses and carefully inspects. "I think it's fine to do nothing," she says.

So, it's settled for now.

MOM, YOU WERE NEVER COOL!

Months after the arbitration is over, in the fall of 2002, I look at Tanya one day and see that her spirit has re-entered her body. She looks like her former self; her blue eyes emanate energy again. Life has begun to feel good once more.

Just in time, too, because Cooper's now a junior in high school and our house is the site of a civil war. He's furious with us about everything: We're too strict, too uptight, too worried, too nerdy. The struggle is intense. We hold the line and set boundaries. He pushes back hard.

Tanya and I retreat to our bedroom and look at each other in desperation. "It's a good thing we love each other," she says, "because if we didn't, divorce would be great. Then, we'd only have to fight with him half the time instead of all the time." She's grinning when she says this.

We decide to take turns being Mom-on-Duty. For much of Cooper's junior year, Tanya is Mom-on-Duty in the early morning, and I don't even come downstairs until he's left for school. If I appear, he "hell hacks" me—our shorthand expression for things like picking a fight or bumping into me, ostensibly by accident, and doing everything he can to be late. He argues with Tanya, too, but reluctantly does what she says.

Cooper decides to join the wrestling team, and for the first time in his life, he says, "I only want one mom for these matches."

"When do you think you'll be *proud* of the fact that you have two moms?" Tanya asks.

"I don't know, probably in about two more years," he says with a certain amount of insight. (Exactly two years later, in the fall of 2004, while in college in Iowa, he'll write a paper on gay marriage, proudly coming out as a kid with two moms.)

"Are you getting homophobic on us?" we tease.

"No, Mom. You don't understand the wrestling environment. It's really macho. My coach thinks I'm a wimp because I have a therapist. They don't believe in things like that."

"You want help with this?" I ask.

"No," he says. "I'll handle it." In his own non-confrontational way, he changes his therapy appointment to a time that doesn't require him to leave practice early.

In response to Cooper's request for one parent at wrestling, I nominate Tanya. Wrestling means lots of weekend mornings at 5 or 6 a.m., when I would prefer to be sleeping. I remind Tanya that she can revert to her wacky blond Texan persona to get by, but that I wouldn't have a prayer. I'm the more obvious lesbian. Fortunately, she accepts my nomination and I sleep.

"I tell you what," Tanya says when she returns from the first tournament. "Cooper got it right. There is *no way* it would have been okay to have two moms at this match." She describes a testosterone-driven event in which parents from the other team yelled things like: "Kill him." "Slam him!" "If you lose, don't bother coming home tonight." She's convinced that these were not hyperbolic, that the parents meant much of what they yelled. Tanya, who's never afraid of *anything*, actually asked the coach to walk her to her car because Cooper's team won and she was worried about getting harassed by the losing team's parents.

When I finally attend a match, I see my son rolling around on a mat, getting thrown around, sweating and red-faced. People scream.

Hands and bodies slam on mats. Whistles blow. I watch, wince, look away, look back. When he wins his match, he's red, sweaty and grinning, and I'm worn out.

Sometimes when Cooper gets angry with us, he goes on the attack. "It's your fault that I worry so much," he says. "You worry, so I worry." If we don't bite, he escalates.

"I wish you were like Anthony's parents. They let him do what he wants. He doesn't have a curfew. Why are you so uptight?"

"Mom, you were never cool!" he yells on another occasion. "You don't know what cool is."

One day, he really goes for it. "My life would have been fine if I'd had a father!" he yells.

The first time he does this, I feel wounded. I buy right in: What have I done? My boy is suffering. It must be my fault, I think.

Finally, after he tries this ploy a few times, I've had enough. "Call me crazy!" I yell back. "But I thought if you had two parents who loved you, and stayed together because they loved each other, and earned enough to take care of you and feed you and give you a few of the nice things in life, you'd be *ahead* of the majority of kids in the world. Half the kids in this country are raised by divorced parents or single parents or grandparents. It didn't occur to me that the gender of your parents would matter that much. I'm sorry, but this is how your life is and you need to get over it and quit whining."

For the moment, he shuts up and just glares at me.

"I actually hate him right now," I say to Tanya after one of these fights.

"We just have to get through this," she says.

"I tell you what. I had no idea it was going to be this difficult. If people actually knew how hard it is to raise a kid, they'd never *have* one." I don't have to tell her that I'm glad we did it. I know she knows. I'm just sick of having to out-macho him.

We see most of our friends, gay and straight, struggling with their teenagers. Some are successful, some aren't. Some kids get sent off to boarding school. Some kids drop out of high school. Some kids go to boot camp. Some kids do well in school but are nervous wrecks. Some get into drugs and alcohol. And some seem just fine. I wonder how that happened.

We carry on. There are rare moments of sweet connection, but it's mostly just difficult. I even have moments when I actually wonder, *way* in the back of my mind, if my former law partner was right: Maybe lesbians shouldn't raise boys. But then I do a reality check. The heterosexuals I know aren't doing any better than *we* are.

In the midst of this drama, Tanya's nephew Chip gallops in from Texas for a visit.

"I'd like to stay out here longer," he tells us after a few days.

"We've got an extra room. Why not stay with us a few weeks?"

Soon, he's settled into our attic. Chip is in his midthirties, a carpenter with a pickup truck, tough, clean and sober, sweet, and a guy's guy. Cooper adores him and Chip adores us. He treats us respectfully and demands that Cooper do the same. Aah, a Top Dog!

Cooper and Chip spend lots of time talking in the attic. Who knows what they talk about? Guy stuff, we figure. They go to movies. They ride around in Chip's pickup.

The weeks stretch into months. Chip helps us with deferred maintenance on our house: painting, stucco work, termite work. At our little cabin on the Russian River, he builds fences and interior walls. On Tanya's fiftieth birthday, the four of us go up to the river and build a platform for a bed in an outbuilding, which we dub the Man Shack. The guys hang out there, and we hang out in the main cabin, which is only four hundred square feet.

When we run out of work, Chip helps our friends, and soon,

he has a little business going. By the time he finally moves back to Texas during Cooper's senior year, peace has been restored to our household.

In June of 2004, Cooper graduates from high school. We throw him a party in our backyard on a warm, sunny Sunday afternoon. Our back porch fills with folks who've known him all his life. So many people want to celebrate that they spill out into the backyard. We drink wine and beer and eat good food. He's beaming. We're proud. It feels like a huge accomplishment to all of us.

In August, he gets ready to leave for Cornell College, a small, liberal arts school in Iowa known for its one-course-at-a-time curriculum. Since it's in the middle of nowhere, we give him my Forester so that he can get to places like Iowa City and Cedar Rapids from the small town where his college is.

Chip flies out from Texas to make the drive with him. They load the car with clothes, camping gear, pillows, books, and bedding, and drive off in the early morning, heading east.

And to my utter shock, I feel my heart being torn out. Who knew? I thought empty nest syndrome happened to stay-at-home moms whose whole lives revolved around their kids. Not to *me! Why didn't anyone prepare me?* Here I am, wandering through the house, seeing reminders of him everywhere. I go into his room just to breathe his scent—cigarettes (unfortunately), incense, shampoo.

Tanya and I go to Calistoga to soak away our blues. I buy a journal at the bookstore and write, "I'm ambushed by feelings I never imagined, as my son moves through time zones away from me. My heart aches. Soon he'll be in an eleven-by-fourteen-foot room with a boy named Erik from Philly."

When we get home, I write: "Tears come unbidden at unpredictable times. Home for lunch. Empty kitchen table. Three days ago it was covered with Triptiks, lists of things to get, lists of things to take. It's bare now except for the yellow pad I write on and my empty yogurt cup. I restrain the impulse to call."

The next day, I write: "Every time I get my keys, I feel like something's missing. Then I remember—Cooper has my car key. It's his car now."

A few nights later, I write: "The house creaks in the middle of the night. Is that Cooper coming home? With a start, I realize that he's not here anymore."

But slowly, ever so slowly, Tanya and I adjust. We get used to Cooper being gone. We eat when we want to. Have popcorn and broccoli for dinner. Go to movies on the spur of the moment. Suddenly, there's so much extra time!

WE ARE FAMILY

When we chose Cooper's donor, we intentionally picked a man who was willing to be identified when Cooper was eighteen. As he grew up, it was assumed he'd decide at some point to meet his father. The only question was when.

Early in his first year of college, he was ready and contacted the sperm bank for information. He was told that they needed to get the contract governing the meeting drawn up by their lawyer. It turns out that Cooper was their first donor-inseminated child to be ready to look up his father.

As we await the contract, Cooper telephones us. "Mom, I just got a call from some people who want to put me in a documentary," he says, calling from his dorm in Iowa a few months after his arrival for his first year of college. "It's about kids raised by two moms." I flash on the email about the film project that I'd sent him months earlier. I didn't realize that Cooper had responded. Now he's been selected by the filmmakers to be in "My Parents Are Gay" on MTV's True Life.

"I think they're interested because I told them I'm about to find my father," he says.

The documentary, about Cooper's first contact with his father, follows our family as we drive across the Bay Bridge to the sperm bank to get the name and contact information of Cooper's father and a half-brother whose mother used the same donor.

There is a sweet clip of Cooper's first call to his father from his dorm in Iowa, followed by a cut to Tanya and me in our kitchen in Berkeley, where we anxiously wait for him to call after they hang up. The camera captures the excruciating passage of time, and our euphoria when Cooper finally calls.

"He says he wants to help me any way he can," Cooper says. "And he wants to meet me whenever I'm ready. He was really nice to me."

Tanya and I burst into tears, a mixture of joy and tremendous relief. It's only *after* Cooper and his father, Stephen, talk that I allow myself to seriously imagine all the ways this experience could have been horrible: his father could have been dead, or mean, or in jail, or a drunk. Worst of all, he could have been completely dismissive and uninterested in meeting Cooper.

I give a little prayer of thanks to the secretary at the sperm bank who pointed to his name when we were down to our final three choices.

Just after Christmas over a year later in 2005, Cooper's on winter break from his sophomore year in college and we're all in Portland, Oregon. Tanya and I are pacing around Pam and Steve's house, waiting for Cooper to return. Pam is my old law school friend and Steve is the sweet man she married during our second year.

This morning, Pam dropped Cooper off at a nearby restaurant for breakfast with his father, Stephen. It's their first face-to-face meeting and he's been gone for hours, through both breakfast *and* lunch.

The doorbell finally rings. Pam opens the door and Cooper stands in the entry next to Stephen. Huge grins across white teeth, long, thin noses, olive skin, short brown hair. Handshakes, hugs, many smiles, laughter, joyful hearts. I look at the two of them. "I can't believe it," I say. "You look alike!"

"You think so, Mom?" Cooper is radiant, bobbing his head back and forth from his mothers to his father.

Pam leads us into the family room, and we chatter away about things I will later forget. But what I *will* remember is how connected I feel to Stephen, as if he'd been part of the family all along. Our intention to have our family be Tanya, me, and Cooper is already a thing of the past.

"I forgot to tell my wife that I donated sperm," he says. "So, we've just gotten married, and we're on our way out of town for a romantic weekend, and I say to her, 'I've got something to tell you.' She looks at me expectantly, that puppy-dog look. You'll see exactly what I mean when you meet her. I told her that I got a letter from a lawyer, return receipt requested, and that I almost didn't accept it at the post office because I thought it might be from my ex-wife. But the guy at the post office said I should take it. 'Why not?' he said. So, I did. I opened it right there in the post office. It was from a lawyer for the sperm bank and said that I have a son from when I donated sperm in 1985 and that my son wants to meet me."

We're all laughing, doubled up—Tanya, me, Cooper, Pam and Steve.

Stephen goes on. "Kathy has been great about me having kids, even when I told her there could be five more donor kids besides Cooper who might want to contact me! She's as excited as I am."

We blab on. We discover that both Stephen's mother and my mother were born on exactly the same day, April Fool's Day 1920. And they are both named Ellen, although my mother goes by her first name, Judy.

"My mother lives south of here," Stephen says. He tells us that he doesn't have biological children except through donating sperm. Cooper will be his mother's first grandson.

"I went down to see my mother on Christmas Day," Stephen continues. "I put the MTV documentary on her TV, and as soon as she saw Cooper, she said, 'That's your son, isn't it?' She's so excited."

Tanya says, "You guys should go see your mother, Stephen." We make a date to have dinner with his wife Kathy that night, and Cooper and Stephen decide to drive to Corvallis to see his new grandmother the next day.

Tanya and I are filled with emotion, relieved that we like Stephen and that he's being so wonderful with Cooper. The intensity of the first meeting is so exhausting that we fall into a deep sleep the moment we go to bed.

The next night, Cooper and Stephen take off in Stephen's Mazda sports car to introduce Cooper to his new grandmother. Tanya and I plot out how long it should take them to drive from Portland to Corvallis in Friday afternoon rush hour traffic, on New Year's weekend, in the middle of an enormous, raging storm that's causing floods all over the Northwest. We figure they should be back to the house by 11:00 p.m. at the latest.

At midnight, I roll over in bed and look at the clock. "Should we check on them?" I ask Tanya.

"No," she says. "Leave them alone." She's always less worried than I am.

At 1 a.m., I say to Tanya, "I don't care what you think, I'm calling." Cooper answers his cell phone after the first ring. "Don't worry. We're out front talking."

At 2 a.m., Cooper walks right into our bedroom without knocking. "I can't believe it. I've never met *anyone* who totally understands me. But, you know what? He understands everything about how *my* brain works because *his* brain works the same way. All these years I've thought something was wrong with me. I thought I was doing something wrong. But, you know what, this is just *how I am*. I don't know if this is a good thing or a bad thing."

I sit up. "How could this be bad, Cooper? Stephen is wonderful: he's sweet, smart, has a good life, a job he likes, a wonderful wife. He's figured out how to deal with a lot of the things you struggle with, and his life is working great."

He looks at me as if this is a revelation. "You're right, Mom. Okay, I'm crashing."

"Before you go, how was your grandmother?"

"We called her before we got there, so she knew we were coming. It's good we didn't surprise her. She had to take some pills to calm down her heart. I walked in the door and said, 'Hi, Grandma,' and she went nuts. Mom, I know I have half your genes, but right now, it feels like they all came from Stephen."

We lie in bed. I think about our sweet son and his sweet father and feel so grateful that Stephen is the person he is. I'm a little stunned at how similar they are. I'd always thought nurture was more important than nature, but this makes me wonder.

Tanya's groggy, half-awake, half-asleep, but I can tell that all the genetic conversation is discombobulating her a little, too. She's a person who had no qualms about being the non-biological mom. When we were deciding who would have a child first, I told her that I didn't think I'd handle the non-bio mom role very well. I felt too insecure. Besides age, this was an important consideration in our decision for me to go first. And until now, biology just hasn't seemed that important. With these thoughts rumbling around, I fall sound asleep.

The next summer, when Cooper is home from college on break, the three of us are invited to discuss the MTV documentary when it's played as part of Piedmont's Diversity Film Series. We've seen the film a number of times, but this time it's on a big screen. The audience is a mixed crowd of about fifty people. The film ends and we're up on stage with a microphone.

"Why did you do the documentary?"

I answer. "A friend of mine sent me an email about the filmmakers looking for kids raised by lesbians. I figured it was Cooper's choice and sent the email to him, thinking he wouldn't be interested. But he was."

"What was it like having them around filming your life?" someone asks.

"You get used to it," Tanya says. "The first day was intense, but after that, we didn't notice that much."

"Have you met your father yet?"

"Yes. Last New Year's," Cooper answers.

"What was it like?"

"Awesome," Cooper beams. "I don't have words for it."

"How has it affected you?"

I couldn't wait for his answer.

"Well, I'd say I'm much more self-accepting," Cooper says.

I watch him holding the microphone, fielding deeply personal, thoughtful questions with an ease I wouldn't have imagined. He's calmer and more grounded than ever.

Someone addresses me: "I notice that you call him 'father' instead of 'donor.'"

I have a strong reaction to this question. Something about the word "donor" feels dehumanizing to me. Stephen is so much more than just a "donor." I realize it's unusual that we call him "father," but it feels just right.

Knowing the intensity of my emotions on this topic, I hand off the microphone to Tanya, who will be gracious and funny. "When we had Cooper, there was no lesbian mom handbook that told us how we were supposed to act." She's laughing. The audience laughs. "When Cooper was little and asked how come he didn't have a dad, we said, 'Everyone has a dad. Some dads are part of the family and help raise you. Some dads aren't. Your dad gave us the seed so that we could have you. He's a good man, but we don't know him. When you're grown, you can meet him.'"

"Did it bother you, Cooper, not to have a father?"

"Well, I didn't think about it much until I was fifteen or sixteen, and then I really wanted to know who he was."

"In fact," Tanya says, "when he was about eight, we asked him if he missed having a father and he said, 'No way, dads give more time-outs.'" More laughter.

"Did you two moms feel anxious or threatened about meeting him?"

"Everyone asks this question," I say. "Like somehow we'll be displaced. But once we knew Stephen was wonderful, we were fine. It's been a good thing."

Which isn't to say there wasn't a moment when Tanya wondered where she fit into the conversation, with all the talk about how genetically similar Cooper and Stephen are. She briefly got off-balance those first few nights, feeling insecure about her role, but it was short-lived. She's Cooper's mother, and in that conviction, we've never wavered and, more importantly, neither has Cooper.

Later, when I have occasion to ask Cooper what was the most important thing that has happened to him in his life, he thinks for a while and then says, "Probably meeting my father."

GIVE THANKS

It's a warm fall day in October, a few months after the end of chemo. I love walking into the Stanford Cancer Center with my hairlets and a bit of energy.

"Let me see what I can remember about Ms. Reaves from memory," Dr. Colevas says as he walks into the treatment room with a student doctor.

"Martina," I say. "It's Martina." I can't believe after all we've been through that he's still so formal!

"Okay," Dr. Colevas says. And then he recites my medical history, fairly accurately listing the three surgeries, the seven weeks of radiation, the four months of chemo. "And how are you today?"

"Pretty good. I still have those little spots on my neck," I say, pointing, "but they haven't grown."

He checks, and then says, "I'm going to do a little surgery." I hold my breath. Tanya and the student doctor peer over his shoulders as he works. I don't feel a thing. "There, it's draining," he says. "They're just little cysts."

I want to both laugh and cry. I've been watching these spots for the last four months. In August when I saw Dr. Colevas, he just said to keep an eye on them, that he didn't know what they were. Every day, like it or not, they were there in the mirror. Little white dots that looked *just* like the spots on my neck last January when my surgeon said I only had months to live.

All this anxiety and it was only cysts! I think about all the time I wasted worrying.

In early November, the doorbell to our home rings. I rush to open the door for Leann, Stephen, and his wife Kathy. Stephen and Kathy are in Berkeley for their annual visit and staying with Leann.

When we got home from meeting Stephen for the first time, we had lunch with Leann and described Stephen and his wonderful Kathy to Leann. Leann suddenly got pale and quietly asked, "What are their last names?" When we told her, she grinned. Kathy is one of Leann's best friends from childhood. What are the chances?

We're all crammed in our cozy kitchen, just barely out of our jammies, in sweats and slippers. No bras. No showers. No formalities. That's how it is with family. Somehow, magically, we were connected to Stephen and Kathy from the beginning, without all the years and years of developing intimacy like one does with new friends.

We sit around our kitchen table, catching up. About Kathy's son, who's a senior in college doing environmental work. About Leann's son Jake, one of Cooper's closest friends. About Cooper and Hayley, who are still asleep in the backyard cottage.

Tanya has made bran muffins with apricots, walnuts, and grated apples. We devour them hot, fresh from the oven, with apricot jam.

"The good thing about having your father appear when you're older," Stephen says to Cooper when he finally wakes up, "is that I'm here at just the right time to teach you about wine." He and Kathy take Cooper and Hayley to the wine country for the day and they all come home for dinner bearing gifts. Even Cooper, who's generally incredibly frugal, bought a few bottles.

—

Later that month, our friend Pam arrives for The Purge. Some of the aftermath of cancer is getting back into your life again, taking care of all the things you ignored while you were sick, including the things you ignored for years!

During a visit with Pam and Steve in July, Tanya confided that she was overwhelmed with what she still had to do to organize her home office from closing her law practice years ago. She brought furniture and office items home as she closed her office, but nothing ever got organized or sorted. This led to a conversation about the attic, which the rats had taken over this time last year. Though we finally won that battle after many months of Tanya's patient work, the mess from the rats remains.

Pam lit up. "I can do this. Pick a week and I'll come down and help you."

Pam is the most organized person I've ever known. In law school, she had neat little lists of chores, homework, work-related tasks, finances. She knows both of us intimately—me from our years of being friends through law school, studying for the bar exam, work, and life; Tanya from working with her for five years. She knows how we think.

Pam was one of the folks who moved us into our house in 1986, when I was in the hospital with pneumonia during my first round of cancer. Everything got packed and moved without help from Tanya and me and with none of the usual sorting and organizing that accompanies a move. When I came home from the hospital to our new house, it was already set up.

Now our house is filled with stuff from Tanya's law office, stuff from my mediation business, stuff that's accumulated over the years we've lived here, stuff we can't bear to get rid of but don't need, and stuff we don't notice anymore because it's been here so long. Not to mention all the stuff that got moved into the house in 1986 when we were concentrating on cancer and not sorting things out. Much too much stuff.

Pam sweeps in and takes over. She surveys everything except the basement, which we agree not to show her for fear it would put her over the edge. Tanya's office looks like it's been ransacked. In the kitchen, the shelf by the phone is piled with papers, tools, cups with pens and pencils, a heating pad, Netflix mailers, and what can only be described as miscellaneous junk. My office is a bit more organized, which is to say that the junk is piled neatly, but it's definitely not serene.

"This is not the Tanya and Martina I know," she says. "I remember when every surface was clean, except a beautiful pot sitting in just the right spot." That seems long ago to me. I don't remember those people.

"We have lots to do," Pam says. "We're gonna start with Tanya's office."

Tanya and Pam tear into the large office closet. Tanya's on a ladder, passing things to Pam who's putting them in piles: recycle, shred, save, trash, move somewhere else, Goodwill.

Here are the things they ask me about: Four batches of leftover stationery from my mediation practice, all with different addresses: recycle. Pottery shards in a shoe box that our neighbor Peter collected in Palestine after World War II just before he immigrated to the States: save. A Teenage Mutant Ninja Turtle still in its plastic container from the shelf where we store items for presents: save to give to Cooper this Christmas as a joke. Piles of recycled files available for re-use: stack. There's much, much more, but I'm spared from having to make decisions about any of it because it belongs to Tanya.

Five-foot tall stacks fill the living room and I take them away to their destinations: the Salvation Army, the street corner, shredding, recycling. Each night we work until 10:00 or 10:30, although I take frequent naps. Pam and Tanya stop for treats: margaritas daily, made according to the Zuni Café recipe, which can't be beat. I refrain from the alcohol, but nibble on some marijuana chocolate chip cookies. We laugh, work hard, blab.

By the time Pam leaves, we're utterly exhausted and our house is calm, uncluttered. Each room has been touched, organized, put together the way we want it, pleasing to the eye and functional.

On Thanksgiving, we're sitting around the kitchen table after having stuffed ourselves with Thanksgiving dinner at Hotel Mac (nobody wanted to cook this year), followed by pecan pie and pumpkin pie and oodles of whipped cream at our house. There are eight of us: my mother, Tanya's mother Laura, Tanya, Cooper, Hayley, Tanya's sister Jimmie Lee, our great-niece Grace, and me.

My mother opens a large paper bag. "Here we go again," I say, rolling my eyes and laughing.

"Now don't make fun of me," my mother says, goading us on. A fanatic recycler since the 1960s, she often brings things she no longer wants to hand out at family gatherings. She starts taking items one by one out of her bag.

"Who wants this?" she asks as she tells a story about each contribution.

"Mom, we just purged our house," I say, laughing. "We don't need any more stuff."

"Just wait," she says.

The list of items in the bag is truly amazing:

Dried roses from flowers that were sent when my father died in 2001. I actually want these for the ritual Aama Bombo prescribed, which I'm planning for Saturday night.

A candle in the shape of an owl. Cooper gave it to my mother when he was nine, one of the first presents he ever selected by himself. "I can't have candles in my place, you know," Mom says. "They're worried about fire." Cooper takes the owl candle and a second candle the color of spring grass.

"Don't y'all remember what your mother brought to recycle at

Easter?" Tanya's sister says to me. "It was ham juice in a zip lock bag, in case someone wanted to use it to cook beans!"

"And that's when you had those new white carpets," Tanya says. We're all laughing, including my mother. She pulls more out of her sack.

Three kinds of toothpicks: colored ones that are round, which I take; flat ones that are plain colored, which someone else takes; and fancy ones with colored paper on the ends for hors d'oeuvres, which Laura takes.

A frog, used to hold the stems when one is arranging flowers. This frog is "special," my mother says, because it looks more like a turtle than a frog, and she got it in Japan. "I think you should put this in the garden," she adds. I take it to nest in my succulents.

A small lock with a key, which Grace grabs as soon as it's out of the bag.

Two stems of millet in a plastic wrapper that my mother used in flower arrangements. Laura wants them to feed her birds. She has a multitude of them flying around her house: parakeets of all kinds. She's so great with birds that one parakeet laid eggs and hatched babies.

A dirty abalone shell. "This will clean up," my mother announces. Laura takes it, too, for her garden.

My mother tries to get someone to take a tin that you'd use to hold Christmas cookies, but nobody will go for it because it's rusted.

"I'll take two of these coasters," Tanya's sister says. And I look up to see that she's referring to the coasters I put on the table for people's teacups.

"No!" I yell. "Those are ours!"

A long, blue scarf emerges from the bag and Grace scoops it up before anyone else has a chance. She wraps it around her neck and poses, red hair loosely hanging over the top.

From the bottom of the bag, another treasure appears. When

Cooper was in the third grade, my mother volunteered in his classroom and then became friends with his teacher, Mrs. Mengel. To this day, they meet each other at Spenger's or Cesar's for martinis or margaritas. Mrs. Mengel saved a lot of her students' work, and she gave this gem to my mother to give to Cooper. It's a card he made with a drawing of a Christmas tree and a menorah. "Dear Mis. [sic] Mengel," he writes. "Thank you for teaching me very good things. Happy hollidays [sic] from Cooper Reaves."

In my writing, the card reads: "Thanks for all your good work. We really appreciate the art, the writing, the fun math. The poetry book he brought home yesterday is lovely! Enjoy your holidays. Martina & Tanya"

I grab this for Cooper's Memorabilia box.

After the Thanksgiving crowd leaves, I begin preparations for the ritual that Aama Bombo prescribed. I'd bought clay at Mr. Mopps, a kids' toy store, to make a clay figure of myself. But the clay is funky and doesn't shape very well.

"I'm just going to go with it," I tell Tanya. "It's a ritual, after all, not an art project." I end up with a figure that looks like a primitive African, Greek, or Mexican sculpture. It's simple, not refined, not what I thought I'd make, but it's what appears. I leave it on a cutting board in the kitchen to dry overnight.

Later, Cooper wakes up from his post-Thanksgiving nap and goes for the leftovers in the kitchen. We bought food at Chow's in Lafayette so we'd have leftovers after we ate out. "This really feels like the holidays," he says. "I'm excited about Christmas." He looks at me, brown eyes clear and vulnerable. "Last year, I was so scared it was going to be my last Christmas with you, Mom."

"Me, too," I say softly.

I have so much to be thankful for.

—

"Wait until you see the sculpture you made for your ritual," Tanya says the next morning. She's coming upstairs because she hears me rumbling around as I wake up.

"What?"

"As you look at it, the right side has a crack," she says. "It's a mirror image of your face."

"Do we have to glue it?"

"No," she says. "It's fine."

When I go downstairs, I look at my doll and see a crack in the spot where my cancer was. Spooky.

I continue my preparations. I'm supposed to have nine kinds of beans for my ritual. I pull things out of the pantry. We've got six kinds of beans. I figure I need three more: kidney, pinto, and black.

I also need nine colors of fabric. "What about the cloth?" I say to Tanya. I'm trying to let this ritual take shape without pushing things. But, in fact, I've been worried about where I'd find all these colors in our house, which is filled with blue jeans and T-shirts, but not a lot of color.

"Let's look in the cedar chest," she says. And there we find a gold mine: all the batiks and tie dies that we made at Camp It Up with Cooper over the years. Finding nine colors is no problem. And the fabrics are joyful, just right.

"What about the tray?" I want to use a wooden one we have in the kitchen, but Tanya says no. She loves that tray.

"Try the basement," she says.

It's the only place in the house that didn't get purged when Pam came. I walk in and there, right in front by the door, is a flat woven basket that Ann gave me that's the perfect size, shape, and material.

It's a weird day, alternately raining and sunny. Tanya and I are standing in the bedroom. She's following up on the house purge by tackling our closet, which has had no attention since I first got sick, meaning no attention for two years, meaning dust balls on the floor with the shoes, and piles of her clothing stacked on top of her shoes. Suddenly, a light rain patters outside and the sun bursts through. The raindrops sparkle as they fall in the backyard. The redwood dances in the wind, and the sun beats into our bedroom. In the corner of the porch, a silvery spider's web shimmers with droplets of rain. "Look," I whisper to Tanya, and we stand there mesmerized until the sun goes behind a cloud.

There's a rainbow out there somewhere.

I go shopping for the beans and then assemble my piece. I dress my doll in all the fabrics. She looks like a peasant, with layers of colorful clothing and a scarf over her head to hold the crack together. I look at her bare white feet hanging out the bottom. My feet are always cold. I put a warm, fuzzy black cloth around her feet. Then, I lay her on top of a batik that Cooper made at family camp. It looks like a big halo, with stars and sky around it. I surround her with the beans and the candle and I'm ecstatic.

When I go to bed, I put her outside, as Aama told me to do, right by the sliding glass door of our bedroom. I'm ready for tomorrow night's ritual.

Saturday arrives clear and breezy. When I've imagined the ritual, I've seen myself below a starry sky on a windy night, spirits moving all around me.

I hardly *ever* read my horoscope. But today I do. It says: "The rug is yanked out unexpectedly, but it needn't be a disaster. Improvise in the moment and you'll land on your feet." A mind like mine can do wonders with this:

There could be an earthquake. Well, if this happens, I'll just walk up to Grizzly Peak and do my ritual there.

Animals could mess with my doll. I climb upstairs and put her on the back deck by the kitchen where I can keep an eye on her.

Our friend Mollie (not the dog) could be sick and then we won't be able to do the ritual on her hill. I can find another spot.

Then, I remember what I've learned about worry—it's a waste of energy—and I go back to my day.

Jill gives me a massage in the attic. Lying on the table, I'm at an angle I've never experienced in this room. The yellow walls glow. Overhead, the skylight is blue with a cloudless sky. But when she turns me on my side, I'm astonished: the second skylight is filled with the arms of the old live oak, silhouetted against the blue sky, the bark like sensuous skin in the late afternoon sun.

At sunset, I suddenly remember that I need flowers for the basket. My only option at this time is the grocery store, where pickings are slim. But way in the back are some happy white daisies with yellow centers. Just right. Standing in line to pay, I notice behind me a tall, voluptuous woman with a bald head. Beside her is a little girl, perhaps four, also bald with little chipmunk cheeks. Probably from prednisone, I think. They are both beautiful.

"How's Ruby today?" the clerk asks as I get ready to leave. Ruby is pirouetting, full of life and energy.

"Good today, thanks for asking," her mom replies.

In the parking lot, I hesitate, glued to the pavement, remembering the kind woman in Calistoga who urged me to be strong when I had just finished chemo. Ruby and her mother walk out of the store, chattering.

"Can I ask a question?" I say.

The woman smiles at me like a bodhisattva. "Of course."

"Is one of you in chemotherapy?"

"Can you guess which one?"

I look at Ruby. "I think it's you, Ruby. I want you to know that I just finished therapy, and my hair is beginning to grow back. It's coming back curly," I say.

"I have a wig," says Ruby.

"I never got one," I say. "But my hair was always straight, and now it's curly. You just never know."

We chat a moment longer and say our goodbyes. I get into my car with my flowers, and halfway home I find tears streaming down my cheeks. What an amazing mother. What an amazing child. My heart splits wide open.

Our friend Mollie has made us a lovely dinner of chickpea soup, salad, and delicious cheese and bread. She has a spot in mind for the ritual overlooking the entire bay, and directs Tanya along the winding streets to the top of a hill outside Berkeley. Lights sparkle everywhere below the expanse of sky. Yesterday's rain has left the air crisp, clean, and cold.

But despite the beauty, as I prepare, I feel uncomfortable. Anxiety ripples through me. The spot feels too exposed, too available to people to tromp over.

"I can't do it here," I say. "I'm really sorry, but this isn't right." I pick up the basket and flowers and walk toward the car. "Can we look for another spot?" I'm calm, thinking about my horoscope.

Fifteen minutes later, the three of us are standing on a hill behind Mollie's house. Overhead, the sky is dark, cloudless, filled with stars. The moon is a few days from being full, a cold silver lopsided orb. The hills of Tilden Park roll off toward the horizon. Around us huge trees reach up and whoosh in the wind. It's a wild night. This feels just right. I improvised and landed on my feet!

I walk down a path, lay my basket under a tree in the pine needles on the ground, and arrange the flowers around it. Tanya and Mollie wait up the hillside while I say my prayers. I'm too shy to do it in front of them. When I'm done, I rejoin them and Tanya goes down to the spot. Mollie and I can hear her chanting when the wind rises up from the canyon. When she's done, I return, chant more meditations, blow out the candle, and we're done.

I feel ready to begin a new chapter, to move into the next phase of my life and whatever it brings.

LESS THAN ONE PERCENT

It's March of 2010, eight months after my last chemo treatment. I'm better, at least better enough for Tanya to be gone for a long period of time. And she is gone—to Texas to help her father, Nelson, who's in the hospital with pneumonia. The phone rings and I run for it. "He's dying," Tanya whispers.

Tanya sleeps on a cot by her father's bed in the dreary hospital, helping the rest of the family begin to accept what's coming. My presence in the hospital would not be welcome. Nelson and his wife believe that Tanya and I are sinners, but they can ignore this fact when I'm not there with Tanya to remind them.

I consider sending flowers, but what I really want is to lighten Tanya's load. I wander through the house. I could organize her chaotic office, which is a mess again, despite the purge with Pam last year. But she'd never find anything if I did the rearranging. I peer outside; it's too waterlogged to work in the garden. Upstairs, the house is fine.

Then it hits me. I change into my work clothes and descend to the basement. Each step increases my dread. I open the flimsy door, duck my head, and step across the threshold onto gravel. The basement is cool, dank, otherworldly. Insulation hangs from the low ceiling. Little vents along the side of the house barely circulate the stale air.

The basement has always been Tanya's territory. Organizing it has been on her to-do list for years. The truth is, I haven't been down here in almost three years except the time I grabbed the basket for my ritual.

Slowly, as I survey the room, my eyes adjust. Oh my god! Rat traps lie on bookshelves, on boxes of tax documents, in dusty corners, with old cheese shriveled up and crumbly. Stacks of file boxes, with labels from Tanya's law practice and my mediation business, practically scrape the low ceiling. Collectibles from Cooper's life line one wall: paintings, a white plaster sculpture of an open zipper that's four feet tall and almost glows in the dingy light, his snowboard and associated paraphernalia, boxes labeled "Report cards, essays, and diplomas" and "Memorabilia."

There's more: Tanya's grandmother's sewing machine. I pull out a drawer and find spools of thread that must be well over a hundred years old. Tanya's multitude of tools, screws, nails, paints, brushes, extra tiles from jobs in two bathrooms and the front porch. I discover my sculpture tools, an antique trunk I've never been able to part with since I got it in the 1970s, boxes of yearbooks, letters, and diaries from my school days.

Our history is layered in boxes down here. I retrieve the telephone so Tanya can reach me if she needs to, and delve in.

Day One: I line up all the paint cans in one area; gather the brand-new plastic bins in another. Tanya bought these bins just before I was diagnosed, meaning to organize things down here. She got derailed.

Day Two: I sort through bags filled with screws, nails, tools, sand-paper. Dust and rat turds fall out of every bag.

Tanya calls. Things are bad in Texas.

"I'm going to tell you what I'm doing, even though it was supposed to be a surprise."

"What? Tell me!"

"I'm organizing the basement!"

"I can't believe it!" she says. "Gotta go. Doctor's here."

She may be preoccupied, but at least she knows that I'm helping in some way.

Day Three: I recycle volumes of empty bags and cardboard boxes; throw out a few things that I know we don't need; put all the lawn chairs in one location. The point is to make the basement *look* better when Tanya steps through the door again, even if it's still far from organized.

For over a week, I work in the basement; some days I put in a few hours; some days, I can only handle thirty minutes. I can see why she's been overwhelmed by it.

Every phone call from Tanya is brief. She's distracted, exhausted, stressed, disembodied. Finally, the end is near.

"Shall I come now?" I ask. "I'll hide in the hotel room and be nice to you whenever you come by." Somehow, I'd always assumed I'd go at the end.

"No, stay in the basement. I love it that you're doing that." She laughs, then whispers, "I just need to get through this part. I'm simply enduring."

When I press her, she starts to cry. "You have no idea how it is here. It's like a foreign country where you don't want to be. I can hardly handle it. And I couldn't bear introducing you to all these people who hate us."

When we hang up, my grief overflows, knowing I can't be there by her side.

I pick her up from the airport after the funeral. She's limp with exhaustion. Numb. For several weeks, she simply recuperates. I don't even mention the basement. Then, one day, it seems right to suggest she take a look. I stand at the top of the stairs and listen as she opens the door and flips on the light. There's a moment of silence, and then she yells, "This is incredible!"

Now we're sorting through things so fast that we make a trip to the shredder or the recycler every day. We actually *open* the boxes that we've been moving and re-stacking over the years: old checks, bank statements, utility and water receipts, credit card bills. We seem to have saved *everything*.

And there are some gems, like the receipt from the Altamira in Sausalito, where we went for breakfast after our first night together in 1980. We unearth the draft of the letter I wrote to my ex-husband while we were negotiating our divorce, which says things like, "Despite its problems, I think we had a relatively good relationship. I don't regret my time with you." We discover the letter to Tanya from our boss, Jerry, when he tried to get her to go to EST. We find the receipt from the Miramonte Hotel in Calistoga, where Tanya and another friend took my law school buddies and me after we passed the bar exam; receipts for all our payments to the OB for Cooper's birth; and the information about two crystal brandy snifters that were the first fancy present I ever bought Tanya after I got my first job as a lawyer.

It feels like we're affirming our life together—clearing out the junk, saving the precious. Making sense of what we've been through. Even though my cancer could come back, I'm comforted that at least now Tanya won't be left with all this mess to sort through by herself.

I have another appointment with Dr. Colevas. April 20, 2010, is just over two years since my original diagnosis. In the early morning, rain slaps onto the skylight above our bed; wind rattles against the glass door. I wake up, restless until I can finally get up and declare it morning.

By the time we're ready to go, the sun is peeking out between puffy clouds. Ever efficient, we load seven file boxes into the back of the Subaru and take them to the shredder on our way to Palo Alto.

Dr. Colevas knocks gently at the door and walks in grinning. He's wearing a blue shirt and a red bow tie, looking adorable as usual. The routine poking and prodding and a quick prick with a needle.

"Just scar tissue," he says. "I can't find anything to worry about. You know you're unique, don't you?"

"Sort of," I say, but I'm not really sure what he means by *unique.*

"You're in a category of less than one percent," he says.

It jolts me, this *less than one percent.* For some reason, I'd assumed that lots of folks have treatment like mine followed by a reprieve like I've gotten. Maybe this isn't the case. "You mean I'm supposed to be dead now?" I ask.

"Yes, or you're supposed to have tumors all over that we can see and feel. There's nothing here."

It's true that I've been hoping for a miracle. I've never given up. But this sounds overly optimistic!

"You need to think about long-term health. Colonoscopies and cholesterol. Of course, you have to keep doing all the things you've been doing, because who knows what's worked. If you've stood on your head for five minutes a day for the past two years, keep doing it." He smiles. Then he writes down all the weird remedies as I recall them—the supplements, acupuncture, Chinese herbs, meditation—and I wonder what he really thinks about my strange practices. After he rolls his eyes at homeopathy, I don't even mention Healing Man or Aama Bombo.

Tanya and I float out of the hospital, drive across the Dumbarton Bridge, the water surreal, merging into the hills and sky. We don't talk, except that every once in a while one of us says, "Less than one percent," as if it is a revelation.

Back home, the basement awaits us. We continue our work, but now I'm thinking, we're preparing for life.

When you're supposed to die, a lot of things just don't seem that important. You can hang out in bliss, love your family and friends, ignore your teeth. You can skip learning to text message. Refuse to figure out how to work the new TV and DVR. Ignore your emotional junk. At least most of the time.

By failing to die, I now have to face all of it.

I find myself not knowing what to do. Exhausted, but wanting to be productive. Unable to think clearly. A psychological wreck.

My calendar doesn't seem to understand the change in my health status. It's still clogged with wellness appointments, and of course, I need healthy food, exercise, and a nap every day.

I feel guilty for whining. I'm alive, after all. Shouldn't I be euphoric?

Another autumn comes, two and a half years since my diagnosis and over a year since my last treatment. Medical appointments, bills, budgets, health insurance, and deferred maintenance of my body, my house, and my relationships crowd my days; I feel like I've been busy, but don't have much to show for my efforts, can't even remember how I've spent my time.

Cooper and Hayley break up and he moves into a flat with other twenty-somethings in West Oakland. He continues with his water conservation job and checks in with us less and less.

Tanya and I struggle to deal with our new reality. While I was sick, it was easy to overlook all the small things that didn't work in our marriage. But we find that the years of dealing with her head injury and my cancer have taken a toll. We've been merged for too long, our lives joined at the hip. We work hard in therapy during this period to clean up our psychological houses and our perseverance and loyalty to each other pay off: we emerge into a peaceful loving place with each other, with better communication skills and, most of all, understanding of and appreciation for our differences.

In late October 2010, Tanya and I take our first real vacation in years, meeting Pam and Steve on Kauai. It's the first time in three years that we've dared to plan ahead for a vacation. Holding on to ropes, we hike down a cliff to the beach below our condo. The salt water feels like an elixir. The sun vibrates in my pores. My body feels strong and healthy, and I'm so relaxed, I actually forget to worry.

When we return, I have another check-in with Dr. Colevas. When he sends me away once more, I email the folks on my cancer list to say that I'm going to deep-six the list, that I don't need it anymore. I declare myself well, affirming once again that I'm among the less than one percent.

And ever so slowly, the people around me begin to relax. Cooper finally goes on the trip he was supposed to take when he graduated from college, flying off alone with his backpack to Hawaii, Australia, and Bali.

Ann stops calling every other day, no longer waiting for the other shoe to drop.

I celebrate my sixty-second birthday in February 2011, and a few days later, I hear a plunk at the front door, the clank of metal against metal. Mail drops through the slot onto the rug: letters, catalogs and a poofy manila envelope. The Catholic-girl script on the envelope has a return address in Kenosha, Wisconsin, and I realize that this is the birthday package Maggie mentioned in an email. It's unusual, since we've been friends for almost forty years, and have never given each other birthday presents when we weren't living in the same place.

I tear open the envelope and two pairs of socks fall out. I recognize one pair as the kind of wool socks I buy at REI; the other pair is new, still in the wrapper.

The note says:

"I stole your socks.
They were left somewhere—
on a bench or in my car
after a trip to the baths in Calistoga.
I could have returned them

But I was afraid.
I was afraid it might be all I had of you.
I could not imagine a world without Martina,
and at least
I could have a world with your socks.
I am not afraid anymore.
You can have your socks back.
I wore them.
Happy Birthday
and many more."

Five months later in July, Tanya and I are at Camp It Up, perched on a hill above the Feather River, sitting in lounge chairs in front of our tent cabin in the afternoon shade. It's three and a half years since my original diagnosis and two years since we canceled a trip to camp for the twentieth-year celebration because I was too depleted from chemo.

The wind in the trees sounds like the roar of the ocean. Wave after wave washes through camp. Then suddenly, the wind completely stops, and there's utter silence.

Time slows. A lizard skitters down the grooved red bark of a Ponderosa pine. Leaves make shadows on the tent. Mosquitoes sleep. My body relaxes. My mind drifts with the shifting shadows.

A gaggle of five-year-olds passes my tent, an array of backpacks, colorful T-shirts, baseball caps, tennis shoes, sweat and dust. Their counselor shouts to be heard above the constant chatter. They meander down the hill, and I'm left with the hum of nature: birds chirping, river rushing, flies buzzing.

During cocktail hour, Tanya, our friend Liz, and I visit in the circle of chairs in front of Leann's tent. All of us were part of Camp It Up in the early days, when our kids were young. We come back because it feels so good to be here with our extended "family."

Liz asks how I am.

"These past two years have been harder in some ways than the cancer," I say.

To my surprise, she nods, as if she knows what I mean. "I remember seeing you when you were at the end of treatment," she says. "We had lunch at that Italian place, and you were way too skinny, but your face was radiant. Then I saw you six months later. You'd put on some weight and looked healthy, but your face was harried and you seemed harassed. It made me think about what it might be like getting back into life again."

"I got my miracle," I say, "but life is not a bowl of cherries. I've had to learn how to live again."

Then Liz brings out red and juicy cherries, as if on cue. Leann makes drinks. We talk about our friend Judy Macks, a long-time camper who died last year of breast cancer. People keep feeling her presence at camp, a glance here, a sound there. As usual when I think of someone close to me who has died, the line from Holly Near's song goes through my mind: *It coulda been me, but instead it was you.*

As we reminisce, a monarch butterfly appears. She flutters in on the breeze, the only butterfly I've seen since arriving. She lands on Liz's foot, Leann's hand, Liz's foot again. For twenty minutes, the four of us sit silently. She flits into the woods, over and over, and reappears, alighting on Liz or Leann like a blessing.

I'm amazed to be here, surrounded by people I love, people who love me. I savor every moment.

Floating on an air mattress on the river, body in hot sun, hands in cold water.

A one-year-old boy in a pink tutu, dancing, dancing, dancing in a circle of clapping giants.

Cooper driving up in my mother's ancient Toyota to be greeted by people who've known him since he was four.

Dancing, dancing, dancing with Tanya and Cooper to the Pointer Sisters singing "We Are Family."

The light and dappled shadows.

The bark of Ponderosa pines, like gullied brown skin.

The waves of wind in the treetops.

The rhythm of waking to cool morning air, the chattering, clattering of breakfast, the midmorning lull after kids go to their groups and adults to their classes, the pandemonium of lunch, the afternoon nap as the breeze caresses my body, swimming in the river, skin smooth and cool, pre-dinner blabbing and cocktail parties, dinner, the evening activity—talent shows, dances, plays. And finally, after dark, flashlighting back to the cabin to the hum of bedtime stories.

The feeling that every breath goes deep, that tension has melted away, that I'm connected to Tanya, to Cooper, to my friends, my history, my community, to this landscape, to this earth. And so alive.

EPILOGUE

Almost four years later, on Friday, June 26, 2015, I'm barely awake, sitting on the side of the bed, when the phone rings. It's only 7:15. Who could it be this early in the morning?

I answer, and Cooper ecstatically announces that the Supreme Court has ruled in favor of gay marriage. I check my iPhone and see a text from Mollie: "Congratulations!" Cooper wants to know if he got it right, since he's in his early-morning-getting-ready-for-work stupor and heard it on the radio.

Yes! Tanya has picked up the downstairs phone, and we all whoop and holler, until I come to my senses and realize it's Friday, a workday for Cooper at his new full-time water conservation job, following six long, part-time years. "We gotta hang up," I say. "You don't want to be late for work because of a Supreme Court decision."

Leann calls, in tears about the decision. "It's not like I'll get married," she says. "In fact, I probably won't. But I can't tell you how much freer I feel today."

She was at work when a straight co-worker from a military family came into her office crying. "Have you heard?"

"What?"

"The Supreme Court made its decision, and you *won*. It makes me proud of all those people in my family who have fought for our freedom. Today, it seems worth it all."

I check Cooper's Facebook page and see that he's already got a rainbow across his photo. "I want to hug your parents so much right now," his friend Nicole writes. "Their wedding ceremony was one of the most memorable moments of my life. . . . Everyone deserves to love and be loved."

I am so grateful to be alive to experience this.

I reflect on change:

I remember our concern that the previous owners of our house wouldn't sell it to us because we were lesbians.

I remember how scary it was when I first had cancer and Tanya wasn't recognized as Cooper's legal parent.

I remember how everyone cried when Tanya adopted Cooper and the judge said the three of us were a legal family.

I remember a lifetime of choosing my vacations carefully, concerned about being two lesbians travelling together without a man.

I remember teaching Cooper's teachers how to talk about our family.

I remember the first time I walked down a street holding Tanya's hand.

I remember the many years I *didn't* hold her hand in public for fear that my clients would see me and not want me to be their mediator.

I remember the year we were the *only* lesbian family at Berkeley's family camp at Camp Tuolumne.

I remember the thrill of finding Camp It Up, and the joy of having our straight friends—Bonnie and Paul with their daughter, Perry, Stu and Susan with their son, Alex, Emily and David with Emily's daughters Clea and Alissa—join us there every year.

I remember crying the first time I heard the Camp It Up camp song: "A family is a group of folks who love each other lots."

I remember how unimaginable it was twenty years ago to think the Supreme Court would say that we belong.

—

Life goes on. Health problems come and go. My cancer story is now past tense. I see life's rhythm more clearly: the ups, downs, serene times, hard times, boring times, busy times. I've discovered that this business of living well is simply much more complicated than the business of dying. Who knew? I got a miracle, and now my job is simply to live my life, whatever's left of it, moment by moment, with as much connection and grace as I can muster. Today, I savor the fragrance of the lilies that Tanya cut from the front yard. Their sweet aroma fills our kitchen.

ACKNOWLEDGMENTS

In 2007, I strolled into my first writing class at the UC Berkeley Extension, *Writing Fiction from Life Experience*, taught by Susan Ito. I was absolutely terrified. But by the end, I felt brave enough to sign up for a memoir class that was (safely) on-line. Fortified with a bit of encouragement after that second class, I enrolled in David Schweidel's *Creative Nonfiction* class and fell in love with writing. I've been taking classes from David ever since.

Without David, this book would probably not have come to fruition. With his excellent guidance, I wrote story after story about my life without thinking about where it all would go. The stories poured out of me over the course of three years. One day, David finally told me to print my stories and put them together, that there was a book to be made. At each step in this process, he edited, suggested, and encouraged.

When I thought that I might have a book, I began to ask friends to read it. I want to especially thank the early readers of draft one many years ago. They encouraged me to keep working: Nancy Barash, Christa Donaldson, Susan Elliott, Ann Gonski, Pam Hull, and my always-supportive wife Tanya Starnes.

A very special word of thanks to Carl Kopman and Karen Hunt for all the Tuesday mornings that we've spent together putting words to paper.

During the early stages of editing and rewriting my memoir, I was invited to join the Addison Street Writers Circle. The nine women in this group have been by my side on much of this journey, both reading and giving excellent suggestions. I thank them all: Sue Ezekiel, Karen Grassle, Ruth Hanham, Eleanor Lew, Vivian Pisano, Kate Pope, Anna Rabkin, Maryly Snow, and Linda Sondheimer.

A very special thanks to all the people who have been in David's classes with me over the years, and especially those who read the book: Anna Brown, Karen Hunt, Carl Kopman, and Claudia Marseille.

I thank others who read many or most of the chapters as they were written: Barbara Ridley, Raleigh Ellison, Paul Davis, Alice Feller, Susan L'Heureux, Kathy Moore, Mike Capbarat, and Sunny Vergara.

Thanks also to the people who read the HOPE chapter: Catherine Sharpe (whose hilarious comments should be framed) and Arlene Kostant and friends to whom she sent the piece.

I thank She Writes Press and most especially Brooke Warner for her work with me on the last round of editing and for her generous support and feedback; Samantha Strom, my excellent project manager for this book; and Tabitha Lahr for her beautiful cover.

Thanks also to copyeditor Vicky Elliott and publicists Crystal Patriarch and Tabitha Bailey.

Finally, I thank all the other readers along the way who read and commented on the later drafts. They encouraged me, made smart suggestions, and told me what was missing: Marge Slabach, Dianne Safholm, Mollie Katzen, Leann Gustafson, Christy Shepherd, Marjorie Cox, Shannan Wilbur, Emily Weaver, Janet Smith, William Segen, Marylou Allen, and the women in my girls' club (Arlene Kostant, Dana Curtis, Maude Pervere, Amy Rodney, and Susan Keel). Please forgive me if you read my memoir and your name isn't here. It's not about you, but my sloppy record keeping.

And a huge thanks to Dr. Colevas and all his staff for their hopeful care.

Finally, I thank my wife Tanya for everything and our son Cooper for being his wonderful self.

ABOUT THE AUTHOR

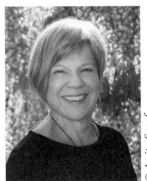

© Anita Scarf

Martina Reaves grew up in a Navy family and lived in thirty-four places before she finally settled in her current home in Berkeley with her wife, Tanya, and their son, Cooper, who now lives in Oakland. She considers living in one place for over thirty years a major accomplishment. A lawyer who hated practicing law, she became a mediator in 1986 and worked with divorcing couples and neighbors with disputes. In 2007, she dropped writing legal documents and began writing fiction and memoir, and she has been at it ever since. She loves creating serenity in her home, gardening, reading, going to plays, and that the music venue Freight and Salvage is five minutes from her home. She thinks eating is wonderful but cooking is boring.

SELECTED TITLES FROM SHE WRITES PRESS

She Writes Press is an independent publishing company founded to serve women writers everywhere. Visit us at www.shewritespress.com.

You Can't Buy Love Like That: Growing Up Gay in the Sixties by Carol E. Anderson $16.95, 978-1631523144

A young lesbian girl grows beyond fear to fearlessness as she comes of age in the '60s amid religious, social, and legal barriers.

Uncovered: How I Left Hassidic Life and Finally Came Home by Leah Lax $16.95, 978-1-63152-995-5

Drawn in their offers of refuge from her troubled family and promises of eternal love, Leah Lax becomes a Hassidic Jew—but ultimately, as a forty-something woman, comes to reject everything she has lived for three decades in order to be who she truly is.

Blue Apple Switchback: A Memoir by Carrie Highley $16.95, 978-1-63152-037-2

At age forty, Carrie Highley finally decided to take on the biggest switchback of her life: upon her bicycle, and with the help of her mentor's wisdom, she shed everything she was taught to believe as a young lady growing up in the South—and made a choice to be true to herself and everyone else around her.

A Leg to Stand On: An Amputee's Walk into Motherhood by Colleen Haggerty $16.95, 978-1-63152-923-8

Haggerty's candid story of how she overcame the pain of losing a leg at seventeen—and of terminating two pregnancies as a young woman—and went on to become a mother, despite her fears.

Hug Everyone You Know: A Year of Community, Courage, and Cancer by Antoinette Truglio Martin $16.95, 978-1-63152-262-8

Cancer is scary enough for the brave, but for a wimp like Antoinette Martin, it was downright terrifying. With the help of her community, however, Martin slowly found the courage within herself to face cancer—and to do so with perseverance and humor.